Health Assessment

made

Incredibly

Visual!™

Lippincott Williams & Wilkins
a Wolters Kluwer business

Philadelphia • Baltimore • New York • London
Buenos Aires • Hong Kong • Sydney • Tokyo

W9-AXQ-580

Staff

Executive Publisher
Judith A. Schilling McCann, RN, MSN

Editorial Director
David Moreau

Clinical Director
Joan M. Robinson, RN, MSN

Senior Art Director
Arlene Putterman

Art Director
Mary Ludwicki

Senior Managing Editor
Jaime Stockslager Buss, ELS

Clinical Manager
Collette Bishop Hendler, RN, BS, CCRN

Clinical Project Manager
Mary Perrong, RN, CRNP, MSN, APRN,BC

Editors
Brenna H. Mayer, Liz Schaeffer, Susan Williams

Copy Editors
Kimberly Bilotta (supervisor), Scotti Cohn,
Karen C. Comerford, Pamela Wingrod

Designer
Lynn Foulk

Illustrators
Bot Roda, Betty Winnberg, Jacqueline Facciolo,
Joseph John Clark, Judy Newhouse

Digital Composition Services
Diane Paluba (manager), Joyce Rossi Biletz

Associate Manufacturing Manager
Beth J. Welsh

Editorial Assistants
Megan L. Aldinger, Karen J. Kirk, Linda K. Ruhf

Design Assistants
Georg W. Purvis, IV; Eoanna Larsen

Indexer
Barbara Hodgson

Derived from *American Gothic,* 1930 by Grant Wood. All rights reserved by the estate of Nan Wood Graham/Licensed by VAGA, New York, NY.

The publishers have made every effort to obtain permission from the copyright holders to use borrowed material. If any material requiring permission has been overlooked, the publishers will be pleased to make the necessary arrangements at the first opportunity.

HAIV010406—040107

Library of Congress Cataloging-in-Publication Data

Health assessment made incredibly visual.
 p. ; cm.
 Includes bibliographical references and index.
 1. Nursing assessment — Atlases. 2. Nursing assessment — Handbooks, manuals, etc. 3. Physical diagnosis — Atlases. 4. Physical diagnosis — Handbooks, manuals, etc. I. Lippincott Williams & Wilkins.
 [DNLM: 1. Nursing Assessment — methods — Atlases. 2. Nursing Assessment — methods — Handbooks. 3. Physical Examination — methods — Atlases. 4. Physical Examination — methods — Handbooks. WY 49 H434 2007]
RT48.H448 2007
616.07'5 — dc22
ISBN13 978-1-58255-985-8
ISBN10 1-58255-985-6 (alk. paper)   2005037928

Contents

Contributors and consultants

Katrina D. Allen, RN, MSN, CCRN
ADN Nursing Faculty
Faulkner State Community College
Bay Minette, Ala.

Barbara S. Broome, RN, CNS, PhD
Associate Dean and Chair,
    Community/Mental Health
University of South Alabama College of
    Nursing
Mobile

**Ellie Z. Franges, RN, MSN, CNRN,
CRNP**
Nurse Practitioner—Neurosurgery
St. Luke's Hospital and Health Network
Bethlehem, Pa.

Virginia D. Lester, RN, MSN, CNS
(INACTIVE)
Assistant Professor
Angelo State University
San Angelo, Tex.

Elizabeth A. Riegle, RN, BSN, MS
Clinical Associate Professor
University of Buffalo (N.Y.), School of
    Nursing

Christie W. Shelton, RN, MSN
Nursing Instructor, Project Director of
    Health Study
Jacksonville (Ala.) State University

Kimberly Such-Smith, RN, BSN, LNC
Legal Nurse Consultant/Case
    Manager/Healthcare Advocate
Nursing Analysis & Review, LLC
Byron, Minn.

**Sandra McSherry Waguespack, RN,
MSN**
Instructor
Louisiana State University Health
    Science Center School of Nursing
New Orleans

Marsha Wamsley, RN, MS
Associate Professor of Nursing
Sinclair Community College
Dayton, Ohio

1 Fundamentals

Ready. Action!

Health history

All assessments involve collecting two kinds of data: *objective* and *subjective.* The health history gathers subjective data about the patient.

Objective data

- Are observed
- Are verifiable
- Include findings such as a red, swollen arm in a patient with arm pain

Subjective data

- Provided by the patient, or "subject"
- Verified only by the patient
- Include statements such as "My head hurts" or "I have trouble sleeping"

Interviewing tips

To make the most of your patient interview, create an environment in which the patient feels comfortable. Also, use the following techniques to ensure effective communication.

> The success of your patient interview depends on effective communication.

- ☑ Select a quiet, private setting.
- ☑ Choose terms carefully and avoid using medical jargon.
- ☑ Speak slowly and clearly.
- ☑ Use effective communication techniques, such as silence, facilitation, confirmation, reflection, and clarification.
- ☑ Use open-ended and closed-ended questions as appropriate.
- ☑ Use appropriate body language.
- ☑ Confirm patient statements to avoid misunderstanding.
- ☑ Summarize and conclude with "Is there anything else?"

Components of a complete health history

Biographical data

Name _____
Address _____
Date of birth _____

Advance directive explained: ☐ Yes ☐ No
Living will on chart: ☐ Yes ☐ No

Name and phone numbers of two people to call if necessary:

NAME	RELATIONSHIP	PHONE #

Chief complaint

History of present illness

_____
_____

Current medications

DRUG AND DOSE	FREQUENCY	LAST DOSE

Medical history

Allergies ☐ Tape ☐ Iodine ☐ Latex ☐ No known allergies
☐ Drug: _____
☐ Food: _____
☐ Environmental: _____
☐ Blood reaction: _____
☐ Other: _____

> Be sure to include prescription drugs, over-the-counter drugs, herbal preparations, and vitamins and supplements.

Childhood illnesses

	DATE

Previous hospitalizations
(Illness, accident or injury, surgery, blood transfusion)

	DATE

Health problems

	Yes	No
Arthritis	☐	☐
Blood problem (anemia, sickle cell, clotting, bleeding)	☐	☐
Cancer	☐	☐
Diabetes mellitus	☐	☐
Eye problem (cataracts, glaucoma)	☐	☐
Heart disease (heart failure, MI, valve disease)	☐	☐
Hiatal hernia	☐	☐
HIV/AIDS	☐	☐
Hypertension	☐	☐
Kidney problem	☐	☐
Liver problem	☐	☐
Lung problem (asthma, bronchitis, emphysema, pneumonia, TB, shortness of breath)	☐	☐
Stroke	☐	☐
Thyroid problem	☐	☐
Ulcers (duodenal, peptic)	☐	☐
Psychological disorder	☐	☐

Obstetric history (females)

Last menstrual period _____
Gravida _____ Para _____
Menopause ☐ Yes ☐ No

> Ask about the patient's feelings of safety to help identify physical, psychological, emotional, and sexual abuse issues.

Psychosocial history
Coping strategies
_____

Feelings of safety
_____

Social history
Smoker ☐ No ☐ Yes (# packs/day _____ # years _____)
Alcohol ☐ No ☐ Yes (type _____ amount/day _____)
Illicit drug use ☐ No ☐ Yes (type _____)

Religious and cultural observances
_____

Activities of daily living
Diet and exercise regimen _____
Elimination patterns _____
Sleep patterns _____
Work and leisure activities _____
Use of safety measures
(seat belt, bike helmet, sunscreen) _____

> Ask about the patient's family medical history, including history of diabetes or heart disease.

Health maintenance history

	DATE
Colonoscopy	
Dental examination	
Eye examination	
Immunizations	
Mammography	

Family medical history

Health problem	Yes	No	Who (parent, grandparent, sibling)
Arthritis	☐	☐	
Cancer	☐	☐	
Diabetes mellitus	☐	☐	
Heart disease (heart failure, MI, valve disease)	☐	☐	
Hypertension	☐	☐	
Stroke	☐	☐	

Review of structures and systems

General health

Neurologic system

Head

Eyes, ears, and nose

Psychological status

Mouth and throat

Neck

Skin, hair, and nails

Endocrine system

Cardiovascular system

Breasts and axillae

Respiratory system

Gastrointestinal system

Hematologic system

Urinary system

Reproductive system

Musculoskeletal system

During the final part of the health history, ask about each body structure and system to make sure that important symptoms weren't missed. Start at the top of the head and work your way down to the toes.

Your patient is vague in describing his chief complaint. Using your interviewing skills, you discover his problem is related to abdominal distention. Now what? This flowchart will walk you through what to do next.

Evaluating a symptom

My stomach gets bloated.

Ask the patient to identify the symptom that's bothering him.

Form a first impression.
Does the patient's condition alert you to an emergency? For example, does he say the bloating developed suddenly? Does he mention that other signs or symptoms occur with it, such as sweating and light-headedness? (Indicators of hypovolemia)

Yes

Do you have any other signs or symptoms?

Take a brief history.

Perform a focused physical examination to quickly determine the severity of the patient's condition.

No

Take a thorough history. Note GI disorders that can lead to abdominal distention.

Thoroughly examine the patient. Observe for abdominal asymmetry. Inspect the skin, auscultate for bowel sounds, percuss and palpate the abdomen, and measure abdominal girth.

Evaluate your findings. Are emergency signs or symptoms present, such as abdominal rigidity and abnormal bowel sounds?

Yes

Intervene appropriately to stabilize the patient, and notify the doctor immediately.

After the patient's condition stabilizes, review your findings to consider possible causes, such as trauma, large-bowel obstruction, mesenteric artery occlusion, and peritonitis.

No

Review your findings to consider possible causes, such as cancer, bladder distention, cirrhosis, heart failure, and gastric dilation.

Devise an appropriate care plan. Position the patient comfortably, administer analgesics, and prepare the patient for diagnostic tests.

Physical assessment

Assemble the necessary tools for the physical assessment. Then perform a general survey to form your initial impression of the patient. Obtain baseline data, including height, weight, and vital signs. This information will direct the rest of your assessment.

Got your tools? Good. Let's get to work!

Assessment tools

- Cotton balls
- Gloves
- Metric ruler (clear)
- Near-vision and visual acuity charts
- Ophthalmoscope
- Otoscope
- Penlight
- Percussion hammer
- Safety pins
- Scale with height measurement
- Skin calipers
- Specula (nasal and vaginal)
- Sphygmomanometer
- Stethoscope
- Tape measure (cloth or paper)
- Thermometer
- Tuning fork
- Wooden tongue blade

ASSESSMENT TOOLS

best picture

Measuring blood pressure

- Position your patient with his upper arm at heart level and his palm turned up.
- Apply the cuff snugly, 1″ (2.5 cm) above the brachial pulse.
- Position the manometer at your eye level.
- Palpate the brachial or radial pulse with your fingertips while inflating the cuff.
- Inflate the cuff to 30 mm Hg above the point where the pulse disappears.

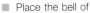

- Place the bell of your stethoscope over the point where you felt the pulse, as shown in the photo. (Using the bell will help you better hear Korotkoff's sounds, which indicate pulse.)
- Release the valve slowly and note the point at which Korotkoff's sounds reappear. The start of the pulse sound indicates the systolic pressure.
- The sounds will become muffled and then disappear. The last Korotkoff's sound you hear is the diastolic pressure.

Tips for interpreting vital signs

- Analyze vital signs at the same time. Two or more abnormal values may provide clues to the patient's problem. For example, a rapid, thready pulse along with low blood pressure may signal shock.
- If you obtain an abnormal value, take the vital sign again to make sure it's accurate.
- Remember that normal readings vary with the patient's age. For example, temperature decreases with age, and respiratory rate can increase with age.
- Remember that an abnormal value for one patient may be a normal value for another, which is why baseline values are so important.

Physical assessment techniques

When you perform the physical assessment, you'll use four techniques: inspection, palpation, percussion, and auscultation. Use these techniques in this sequence except when you perform an abdominal assessment.

> Because palpation and percussion can alter bowel sounds, the sequence for assessing the abdomen is inspection, auscultation, percussion, and palpation.

Inspection

Inspect each body system using vision, smell, and hearing to assess normal conditions and deviations. Observe for color, size, location, movement, texture, symmetry, odors, and sounds as you assess each body system.

Palpation

Palpation requires you to touch the patient with different parts of your hands, using varying degrees of pressure. Because your hands are your tools, keep your fingernails short and your hands warm. Wear gloves when palpating mucous membranes or areas in contact with body fluids. Palpate tender areas last.

Types of palpation

Light palpation
- Use this technique to feel for surface abnormalities.
- Depress the skin ½" to ¾" (1.5 to 2 cm) with your finger pads, using the lightest touch possible.
- Assess for texture, tenderness, temperature, moisture, elasticity, pulsations, superficial organs, and masses.

Deep palpation
- Use this technique to feel internal organs and masses for size, shape, tenderness, symmetry, and mobility.
- Depress the skin 1½" to 2" (4 to 5 cm) with firm, deep pressure.
- Use one hand on top of the other to exert firmer pressure, if needed.

3 Percussion

Percussion involves tapping your fingers or hands quickly and sharply against parts of the patient's body to help you locate organ borders, identify organ shape and position, and determine if an organ is solid or filled with fluid or gas.

Types of percussion

Direct percussion

This technique reveals tenderness; it's commonly used to assess an adult patient's sinuses. Here's how to do it:

■ Using one or two fingers, tap directly on the body part.
■ Ask the patient to tell you which areas are painful, and watch his face for signs of discomfort.

Indirect percussion

This technique elicits sounds that give clues to the makeup of the underlying tissue. Here's how to do it:

■ Press the distal part of the middle finger of your nondominant hand firmly on the body part.
■ Keep the rest of your hand off the body surface.
■ Flex the wrist of your dominant hand.
■ Using the middle finger of your dominant hand, tap quickly and directly over the point where your other middle finger touches the patient's skin.
■ Listen to the sounds produced.

4 Auscultation

Auscultation involves listening for various breath, heart, and bowel sounds with a stethoscope.

Getting ready

■ Provide a quiet environment.
■ Make sure the area to be auscultated is exposed. (Auscultating over a gown or bed linens can interfere with sounds.)
■ Warm the stethoscope head in your hand.
■ Close your eyes to help focus your attention.

How to auscultate

■ Use the diaphragm to pick up high-pitched sounds, such as first (S_1) and second (S_2) heart sounds. Hold the diaphragm firmly against the patient's skin, enough to leave a slight ring on the skin afterward.
■ Use the bell to pick up low-pitched sounds, such as third (S_3) and fourth (S_4) heart sounds. Hold the bell lightly against the patient's skin, just enough to form a seal. Holding the bell too firmly causes the skin to act as a diaphragm, obliterating low-pitched sounds.
■ Listen to and try to identify the characteristics of one sound at a time.

Documentation

Get to know your stethoscope

Your stethoscope should have snug-fitting ear tips, which you'll position toward your nose. The stethoscope should also have tubing no longer than 15″ (38.1 cm) with an internal diameter not greater than ⅛″ (0.3 cm). It should have both a diaphragm and bell. The parts of a stethoscope are labeled below.

Headset
- Ear tips
- Binaurals (ear tubes)
- Tension bar
- Tubing
- Bell
- Stem
- Diaphragm

Chestpiece

take note

Documenting initial assessment findings

Here's an example of how to record your findings on an initial assessment form.

General information

Name __Henry Gibson__

Age __55__ Sex __M__ Height __163 cm__ Weight __57 kg__

T __37°C__ P __76__ R __14__ B/P (R) __150/90 sitting__ (L) __148/88 sitting__

Room __328__

Admission time __0800__

Admission date __1-28-06__

Doctor __Manzel__

Admitting diagnosis:
__Pneumonia__

Patient's stated reason for hospitalization __"To get rid of the pneumonia"__

Allergies __Penicillin Codeine__

Current medications __None__

Name	Dosage	Last taken

General survey

In no acute distress, slender, appears younger than stated age. Alert and well-groomed. Communicates well. Makes eye contact and expresses appropriate concern throughout exam.
— C. Smith, RN

VISION QUEST

Show and tell

Identify the assessment technique being used in each illustration.

1. _____

2. _____

My word!

Unscramble the words at right to discover terms related to fundamentals of assessment. Then use the circled letters from those words to answer the question posed.

Question: Assessment of which body part does not follow the usual sequence?

1. tunicaastolu ◯ _ _ _ _ _ _ _ _ _ _ _ ◯ _

2. divateacub jest _ _ ◯ _ _ _ _ _ _ _ ◯ _ _

3. place inchmotif _ _ _ _ ◯ _ _ _ ◯ _ _ _ _ _

4. aplaintop _ _ _ _ _ _ _ _ ◯ _

Answer: _ _ _ _ _ _ _ _

2
Skin, hair, and nails

Quiet on the set. The assessment is about to begin.

Anatomy

Skin

The skin covers and protects the internal structures of the body. It consists of two distinct layers: the **epidermis** and the **dermis**. **Subcutaneous tissue** lies beneath these layers.

Epidermis
- Outer layer
- Made of squamous epithelial tissue

Dermis
- Thick, deeper layer
- Consists of connective tissue and an extracellular material (matrix), which contributes to the skin's strength and pliability
- Location of blood vessels, lymphatic vessels, nerves, hair follicles, and sweat and sebaceous glands

Subcutaneous tissue
- Beneath dermis and epidermis
- Consists mostly of adipose and other connective tissues

Stratum corneum

Pore of sweat gland

Free nerve ending

Eccrine sweat gland

Hair bulb

Sensory nerve fibers

Autonomic nerve fibers

Artery — — Vein

Hair

Hair is formed from keratin produced by matrix cells in the dermal layer of the skin. Each hair lies in a hair follicle.

Nails

Nails are formed when epidermal cells are converted into hard plates of keratin.

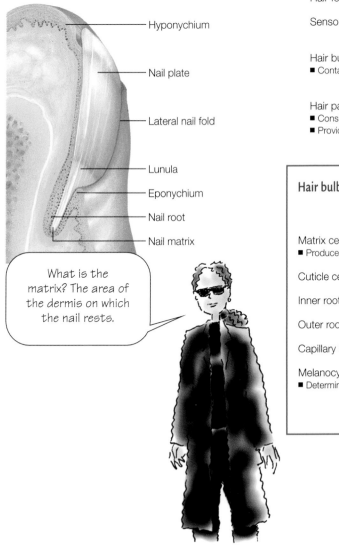

- Hyponychium
- Nail plate
- Lateral nail fold
- Lunula
- Eponychium
- Nail root
- Nail matrix

What is the matrix? The area of the dermis on which the nail rests.

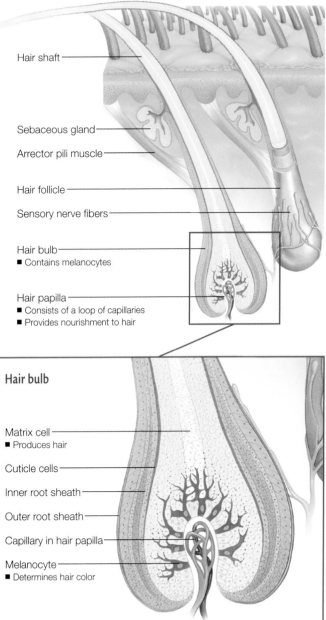

- Hair shaft
- Sebaceous gland
- Arrector pili muscle
- Hair follicle
- Sensory nerve fibers
- Hair bulb
  - Contains melanocytes
- Hair papilla
  - Consists of a loop of capillaries
  - Provides nourishment to hair

Hair bulb

- Matrix cell
  - Produces hair
- Cuticle cells
- Inner root sheath
- Outer root sheath
- Capillary in hair papilla
- Melanocyte
  - Determines hair color

Assessment

Be sure to wear gloves during your examination of the skin, hair, and nails.

To assess the skin, hair, and nails, use inspection and palpation.

Skin

Observe the skin's overall appearance. Then inspect and palpate the skin area by area, focusing on color, moisture, texture, turgor, and temperature.

Color

Look for localized areas of bruising, cyanosis, pallor, and erythema. Check for uniformity of color and hypopigmented or hyperpigmented areas.

Detecting color variations in dark-skinned people

Cyanosis	Edema	Erythema	Jaundice	Pallor	Petechiae	Rashes
Examine the conjunctivae, palms, soles, buccal mucosa, and tongue. Look for dull, dark color.	Examine the area for decreased color and palpate for tightness.	Palpate the area for warmth.	Examine the sclerae and hard palate in natural, not fluorescent, light if possible. Look for a yellow color.	Examine the sclerae, conjunctivae, buccal mucosa, lips, tongue, nail beds, palms, and soles. Look for an ashen color.	Examine areas of lighter pigmentation such as the abdomen. Look for tiny, purplish red dots.	Palpate the area for skin texture changes.

Moisture

Observe the skin's moisture content. The skin should be relatively dry, with a minimal amount of perspiration.

Texture and turgor

Inspect and palpate the skin's texture, noting its thickness and mobility. It should look smooth and be intact.

To assess skin turgor in an infant, grasp a fold of loosely adherent abdominal skin between your thumb and forefinger and pull the skin taut. Then release the skin. The skin should quickly return to its normal position. If the skin remains tented, the infant has poor turgor.

best picture

Assessing skin turgor in an adult

Gently squeeze the skin on the forearm or sternal area between your thumb and forefinger, as shown.

If the skin quickly returns to its original shape, the patient has normal turgor. If it returns to its original shape slowly over 30 seconds or maintains a tented position, as shown, the skin has poor turgor.

Temperature

Palpate the skin bilaterally for temperature using the dorsal surface of your hands and fingers. The dorsal surface is the most sensitive to temperature changes. Warm skin suggests normal circulation; cool skin, a possible underlying disorder.

Normal skin variations

You may see normal variations in the skin's texture and pigmentation. Such variations may include nevi, or moles, and freckles (shown below).

Hair

When assessing the hair, note the distribution, quantity, texture, and color. Hair should be evenly distributed.

Nails

Examine the nails for color, shape, thickness, consistency, and contour. Nail color is pink in light-skinned people and brown in dark-skinned people. The nail surface should be slightly curved or flat and the edges smooth and rounded.

I know you'll have these assessment skills nailed in no time!

Skin abnormalities

Lesions

When evaluating a lesion, you'll need to classify it as primary (new) or secondary (a change in a primary lesion). Then determine if it's solid or fluid-filled and describe its characteristics, pattern, location, and distribution. Include a description of symmetry, borders, color, configuration, diameter, and drainage.

Lesion distribution

Generalized — Distributed all over the body
Regionalized — Limited to one area of the body
Localized — Sharply limited to a specific area
Scattered — Dispersed either densely or widely
Exposed areas — Limited to areas exposed to the air or sun
Intertriginous — Limited to areas where skin comes in contact with itself

Lesion shapes

Discoid

Round or oval

Annular

Circular with central clearing

Target (bull's eye)

Annular with central internal activity

Lesion configurations

Discrete

Individual lesions are separate and distinct.

Grouped

Lesions are clustered together.

Confluent

Lesions merge so that discrete lesions are not visible or palpable.

Dermatomal

Lesions form a line or an arch and follow a dermatome.

outside the norm

Types of skin lesions

Pustule

A small, pus-filled lesion (called a *follicular pustule* if it contains a hair)

Cyst

A closed sac in or under the skin that contains fluid or semisolid material

Nodule

A raised lesion detectable by touch that's usually 1 cm or more in diameter

Wheal

A raised, reddish area that's commonly itchy and lasts 24 hours or less

Fissure

A painful, cracklike lesion of the skin that extends at least into the dermis

Bulla

A large, fluid-filled blister that's usually 1 cm or more in diameter

Macule

A small, discolored spot or patch on the skin

Ulcer

A craterlike lesion of the skin that usually extends at least into the dermis

take note

Documenting a skin lesion

| 4/15/06 | 0845 | At 0820, pt. c/o right shoulder blade pain, 4/10 on a 0-10 scale. A closed, purulent lesion noted in right upper scapular region of back, approx. 1.5 cm x 1 cm, with 3 cm surrounding area of erythema. T 100.2° F. Call placed to Dr. Tomlin's service at 0830. — Angela Kessler, RN |

Vesicle

A small, fluid-filled blister that's usually 1 cm or less in diameter

Papule

A solid, raised lesion that's usually less than 1 cm in diameter

Benign versus cancerous lesions

Lesions may be benign, such as a benign nevus, or mole. However, changes in an existing growth on the skin or a new growth that ulcerates or doesn't heal could indicate cancer or a precancerous lesion.

Benign nevus

- Symmetrical, round, or oval shape
- Sharply defined borders
- Uniform, usually tan or brown color
- Less than 6 mm in diameter
- Flat or raised

Note the differences between benign and cancerous lesions.

Precancerous actinic keratosis

- Abnormal changes in keratinocytes
- Can become squamous cell carcinoma

Dysplastic nevus

- Abnormal growth of melanocytes in a mole
- Can become malignant melanoma

If you suspect a lesion may be malignant melanoma, observe for these characteristics.

Less severe

More severe

Basal cell carcinoma

- Most common skin cancer
- Usually spreads only locally

Squamous cell carcinoma

- Begins as a firm, red nodule or scaly, crusted, flat lesion
- Can spread if not treated

Malignant melanoma

- Can arise on normal skin or from an existing mole
- If not treated promptly, can spread to other areas of skin, lymph nodes, or internal organs

memory board

ABCDEs of malignant melanoma

A = Asymmetrical lesion

B = Border irregular

C = Color of lesion varies with shades of tan, brown, or black and, possibly, red, blue, or white

D = Diameter greater than 6 mm

E = Elevated or enlarging lesion

Common skin disorders

Psoriasis

Psoriasis is a chronic disease of marked epidermal thickening. Plaques are symmetrical and generally appear as red bases topped with silvery scales. The lesions, which may connect with one another, occur most commonly on the scalp, elbows, and knees.

Contact dermatitis

Contact dermatitis is an inflammatory disorder that results from contact with an irritant. Primary lesions include vesicles, large oozing bullae, and red macules that appear at localized areas of redness. These lesions may itch and burn.

Urticaria (hives)

Occurring as an allergic reaction, urticaria appears suddenly as pink, edematous papules or wheals (round elevations of the skin). Itching is intense. The lesions may become large and contain vesicles.

Herpes zoster

Herpes zoster appears as a group of vesicles or crusted lesions along a nerve root. The vesicles are usually unilateral and appear mostly on the trunk. These lesions cause pain but not a rash.

Scabies

Mites, which can be picked up from an infested person, burrow under the skin and cause scabies lesions. The lesions appear in a straight or zigzagging line about ⅜" (1 cm) long with a black dot at the end. Commonly seen between the fingers, at the bend of the elbow and knee, and around the groin, abdomen, or perineal area, scabies lesions itch and may cause a rash.

Once I burrow under the skin, I settle down and make myself comfortable.

Tinea corporis (ringworm)

Tinea corporis is characterized by round, red, scaly lesions that are accompanied by intense itching. These lesions have slightly raised, red borders consisting of tiny vesicles. Individual rings may connect to form patches with scalloped edges. They usually appear on exposed areas of the body.

Pressure ulcers

Pressure ulcers are localized areas of skin breakdown that occur as a result of prolonged pressure. Necrotic tissue develops because the vascular supply to the area is diminished.

> Welcome hither, and learn thee of pressure ulcer stages. As Shakespeare knew, all the world's a stage...

Staging pressure ulcers

You can use pressure ulcer characteristics gained from your assessment to stage the pressure ulcer, as described here. Staging reflects the anatomic depth of exposed tissue. Keep in mind that if the wound contains necrotic tissue, you won't be able to determine the stage until you can see the wound base.

Stage I

- Reddened area
- Epidermis
- Dermis
- Subcutaneous tissue
- Muscle
- Bone

> To blanch, or not to blanch: that is the question. The first sign of a pressure ulcer is a reddened area of intact skin that blanches not. In those with dark skin, warmth, edema, discoloration, induration, or hardness you may spot.

> Double, double, toil and trouble. Marked by partial-thickness skin loss involving the epidermis, dermis, or both is stage II. And superficial though the ulcer be, an abrasion, a blister, or a shallow crater you may see.

Stage II

- Reddened area
- Blister
- Epidermis
- Dermis
- Subcutaneous tissue
- Muscle
- Bone

Stage III

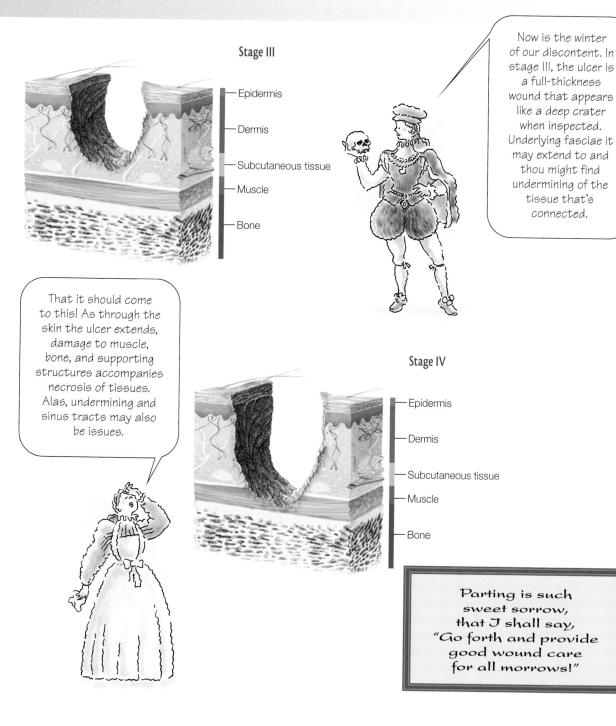

- Epidermis
- Dermis
- Subcutaneous tissue
- Muscle
- Bone

Now is the winter of our discontent. In stage III, the ulcer is a full-thickness wound that appears like a deep crater when inspected. Underlying fasciae it may extend to and thou might find undermining of the tissue that's connected.

That it should come to this! As through the skin the ulcer extends, damage to muscle, bone, and supporting structures accompanies necrosis of tissues. Alas, undermining and sinus tracts may also be issues.

Stage IV

- Epidermis
- Dermis
- Subcutaneous tissue
- Muscle
- Bone

Parting is such sweet sorrow, that I shall say, "Go forth and provide good wound care for all morrows!"

Hair abnormalities

Typically stemming from other problems, hair abnormalities can cause patients emotional distress. Among the most common hair abnormalities are alopecia and hirsutism.

Now "hair" this: Hair abnormalities may be caused by certain drugs or endocrine problems.

outside the norm

Alopecia

Alopecia occurs more commonly and extensively in men than in women. Diffuse hair loss, though commonly a normal part of aging, may occur as a result of pyrogenic infections, chemical trauma, ingestion of certain drugs, and endocrinopathy and other disorders. Tinea capitis, trauma, and full-thickness burns can cause patchy hair loss.

Hirsutism

Excessive hairiness in women, or hirsutism, can develop on the body and face, affecting the patient's self-image. Localized hirsutism may occur on pigmented nevi. Generalized hirsutism can result from certain drug therapy or from such endocrine problems as Cushing's syndrome, polycystic ovary syndrome, and acromegaly.

Nail abnormalities

Although many nail abnormalities are harmless, some point to serious underlying problems. Nail abnormalities include clubbed fingers, splinter hemorrhages of the nail bed, and Terry's nails.

outside the norm

Splinter hemorrhages

Splinter hemorrhages are reddish brown narrow streaks under the nails. They run in the same direction as nail growth and are caused by minor trauma. They can also occur in patients with bacterial endocarditis.

Clubbed fingers

Clubbed fingers can result from chronic tissue hypoxia. Normally, the angle between the fingernail and the point where the nail enters the skin is about 160 degrees. Clubbing occurs when that angle increases to 180 degrees or more.

Normal fingers

Normal angle (160 degrees)

Clubbed fingers

Angle greater than 180 degrees

Enlarged and curved nail

Terry's nails

Terry's nails are characterized by transverse bands of white that cover the nail, except for a narrow zone at the distal end. They're associated with aging and chronic disorders, such as cirrhosis, heart failure, and type 2 diabetes.

Able to label?

Identify the skin structures indicated on this illustration.

1.

2.

3.

4.

5.

Rebus riddle

Sound out each group of pictures and symbols to reveal terms that complete this assessment consideration.

The [ ] + SAL SUR + 😊 of the 🖐 is most 1¢ + SI + TIVE 2 🌡 🪙🪙 + ES.

Answers: Able to label 1. Epidermis, 2. Dermis, 3. Subcutaneous tissue, 4. Hair bulb, 5. Eccrine sweat gland; Rebus riddle The dorsal surface of the hand is most sensitive to temperature changes.

3
Eyes and ears

Aye, aye, matey! I best be gettin' along. They're filming the eye and ear assessment down on Soundstage 3.

Anatomy

Eye

The eyes are delicate sensory organs equipped with many extraocular and intraocular structures. Some structures are easily visible, whereas others can only be viewed with special instruments, such as an ophthalmoscope.

Extraocular structures

The bony orbits protect the eyes from trauma. The eyelids (or palpebrae), lashes, and lacrimal gland, punctum, canaliculi, and sac protect the eyes from injury, dust, and foreign bodies.

- Bony orbit
- Lacrimal gland
  - Pars orbitalis
  - Pars palpebralis
- Upper eyelid
- Lashes
- Lower eyelid
- Lacrimal punctum
- Lacrimal canaliculi
- Lacrimal sac
- Nasolacrimal duct

Eye muscles

- Superior oblique muscle
- Superior rectus muscle
- Medial rectus muscle
- Lateral rectus muscle
- Inferior rectus muscle
- Inferior oblique muscle

Intraocular structures

The intraocular structures of the eye are directly involved in vision. The eye has three layers of tissue:

■ The outermost layer includes the transparent cornea and the sclera, which maintain the form and size of the eyeball.

■ The middle layer includes the choroid, ciliary body, and iris. Pupil size is controlled by involuntary muscles in this region.

■ The innermost layer is the retina, which receives visual stimuli and sends them to the brain.

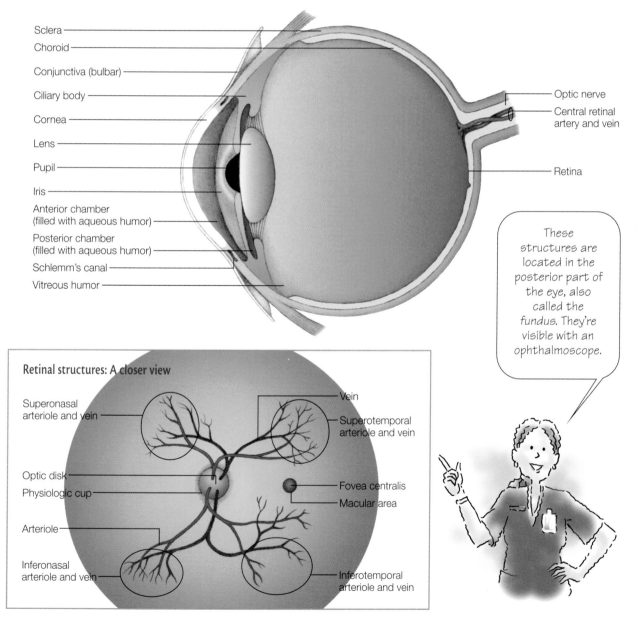

Sclera
Choroid
Conjunctiva (bulbar)
Ciliary body
Cornea
Lens
Pupil
Iris
Anterior chamber (filled with aqueous humor)
Posterior chamber (filled with aqueous humor)
Schlemm's canal
Vitreous humor

Optic nerve
Central retinal artery and vein
Retina

These structures are located in the posterior part of the eye, also called the fundus. They're visible with an ophthalmoscope.

Retinal structures: A closer view

Superonasal arteriole and vein
Optic disk
Physiologic cup
Arteriole
Inferonasal arteriole and vein

Vein
Superotemporal arteriole and vein
Fovea centralis
Macular area
Inferotemporal arteriole and vein

Ear

External ear

The flexible external ear consists mainly of elastic cartilage. It contains the ear flap, also known as the *auricle* or *pinna*, and the auditory canal.

This part of the ear collects and transmits sound to the middle ear.

Middle ear

The *tympanic membrane* separates the external and middle ear. The center, or umbo, is attached to the tip of the long process of the *malleus* on the other side of the tympanic membrane. The *eustachian tube* connects the middle ear with the nasopharynx, equalizing air pressure on either side of the tympanic membrane.

The middle ear conducts sound vibrations to the inner ear.

Inner ear

The *inner ear* consists of closed, fluid-filled spaces within the temporal bone. It contains the bony labyrinth, which includes three connected structures: the *vestibule*, the *semicircular canals*, and the *cochlea*.

The inner ear receives vibrations from the middle ear that stimulate nerve impulses. These impulses travel to the brain, and the cerebral cortex interprets the sound.

Helix

Anthelix

External acoustic meatus

Lobule of auricle

Auditory ossicles
- Stapes (stirrup)
- Incus (anvil)
- Malleus (hammer)

Tympanic membrane (eardrum)

Semicircular canals

Vestibule

Cochlea

Cochlear nerve

Eustachian tube

Assessment

Eyes

Distance vision

To measure distance vision:

👆 Have the patient sit or stand 20′ (6.1 m) from the chart.

✌️ Cover his left eye with an opaque object.

🤟 Ask him to read the letters on one line of the chart and then to move downward to increasingly smaller lines until he can no longer discern all of the letters.

🖐️ Have him repeat the test covering his right eye.

🖐️ Have him read the smallest line he can read with both eyes uncovered to test his binocular vision.

🖐️ If the patient wears corrective lenses, have him repeat the test wearing them.

🖐️ Record the vision with and without correction.

Snellen charts

The Snellen alphabet chart and the Snellen E chart are used to test distance vision and measure visual acuity.

Snellen alphabet chart

Snellen E chart

The Snellen E chart is used for young children and adults who can't read.

Recording results

Visual acuity is recorded as a fraction. The top number (20) is the distance between the patient and the chart. The bottom number is the distance from which a person with normal vision could read the line. The larger the bottom number, the poorer the patient's vision.

Age differences

20/20 In adults and children age 6 and older, normal vision is measured as 20/20.

20/30 For children age 5, normal vision is 20/30.

20/40 For children age 4, normal vision is 20/40.

20/50 For children age 3 and younger, normal vision is 20/50.

Near-vision

To measure near-vision:

Cover one of the patient's eyes with an opaque object.

Hold the Rosenbaum card 14″ (35.6 cm) from the eyes.

Have the patient read the line with the smallest letters he can distinguish.

Repeat the test with the other eye.

If the patient wears corrective lenses, have him repeat the test while wearing them.

Record the visual accommodation with and without corrective lenses.

Rosenbaum card

The Rosenbaum card is used to evaluate near-vision. This small, handheld card has a series of numbers, E's, X's, and O's in graduated sizes. Visual acuity is indicated on the right side of the chart in either distance equivalents or Jaeger equivalents.

Card is held in good light 14 inches from eye. Record vision for each eye separately with and without glasses. Presbyopic patients should read through bifocal segment. Check myopes with glasses only.

DESIGN COURTESY J G ROSENBAUM M D CLEVELAND OHIO

PUPIL GAUGE (mm.)

Confrontation

Test peripheral vision using confrontation. Confrontation can help identify such abnormalities as homonymous hemianopsia and bitemporal hemianopsia. Here's how to test confrontation:

■ Sit or stand directly across from the patient and have him focus his gaze on your eyes.

■ Place your hands on either side of the patient's head at the level of his ears so that they're about 2′ apart.

■ Tell the patient to focus his gaze on you as you gradually bring your wiggling fingers into his visual field.

■ Instruct the patient to tell you as soon as he can see your wiggling fingers; he should see them at the same time you do.

■ Repeat the procedure while holding your hands at the superior and inferior positions.

Does your patient wear glasses or contacts? Remember to test his vision with and without his corrective lenses.

Inspecting the eyes

With the scalp line as the starting point, determine whether the eyes are in a normal position. They should be about one-third of the way down the face and about one eye's width apart from each other. Then assess the eyelids, corneas, conjunctivae, sclerae, irises, and pupils.

Eyelids

Each upper eyelid should cover the top quarter of the iris so the eyes look alike. Look for redness, edema, inflammation, or lesions on the lids.

Corneas

The corneas should be clear and without lesions and should appear convex.

Examining the corneas

Examine the corneas by shining a penlight first from both sides and then from straight ahead. Test corneal sensitivity by lightly touching the cornea with a wisp of cotton.

Irises

The irises should appear flat and should be the same size, color, and shape.

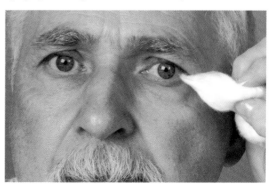

Conjunctivae and sclerae

The conjunctivae should be clear and shiny. Note excessive redness or exudate. The sclerae should be white or buff.

Inspecting the conjunctiva and sclera

To inspect the bulbar conjunctiva, ask the patient to look up and gently pull the lower eyelid down. Then have the patient look down and lift the upper lid to examine the palpebra conjunctiva.

Pupils

Each pupil should be equal in size, round, and about one-fourth the size of the iris in normal room light.

Testing the pupils

Slightly darken the room. Then test the pupils for direct response (reaction of the pupil you're testing) and consensual response (reaction of the opposite pupil) by holding a penlight about 20″ (51 cm) from the patient's eyes, directing the light at the eye from the side.

Next, test accommodation by placing your finger about 4″ (10 cm) from the bridge of the patient's nose. Ask him to look at a fixed object in the distance and then to look at your finger. His eyes should converge and his pupils should constrict.

Grading pupil size

| 1 mm | 2 mm | 3 mm | 4 mm | 5 mm | 6 mm | 7 mm | 8 mm | 9 mm |

Assessing eye muscle function

Corneal light reflex

Ask the patient to look straight ahead; then shine a penlight on the bridge of his nose from 12″ to 15″ (30.5 to 38 cm) away. The light should fall at the same spot on each cornea. If it doesn't, the eyes aren't being held in the same plane by the extraocular muscles. The patient likely lacks muscle coordination, a condition called *strabismus*.

Cardinal positions of gaze

Cardinal positions of gaze evaluate the oculomotor, trigeminal, and abducens cranial nerves and the extraocular muscles.

Ask the patient to remain still while you hold a pencil or other small object directly in front of his nose at a distance of about 18″ (45 cm).

Ask him to follow the object with his eyes, without moving his head.

Move the object to each of the six cardinal positions shown, returning to the midpoint after each movement.

Right superior (RS)	Left superior (LS)
Right lateral (RL)	Left lateral (LL)
Right inferior (RI)	Left inferior (LI)

Note abnormal findings, such as nystagmus (involuntary, rhythmic oscillation of the eyeballs) or amblyopia (failure of one eye to follow an object).

Examining intraocular structures

Before beginning your examination, ask the patient to remove his contact lenses (if they're tinted) or eyeglasses. Then darken the room to dilate the patient's pupils and make your examination easier. Ask the patient to focus on a point behind you.

Set the lens disc at zero diopter, hold the *ophthalmoscope* about 4″ (10 cm) from the patient's eye, and direct the light through the pupil to elicit the red reflex. Check the red reflex for depth of color.

Adjust the lens disc so you can focus on the anterior chamber and lens. Look for clouding, foreign matter, or opacities.

The ophthalmoscope

The ophthalmoscope allows you to directly observe the eye's internal structures. Use the green, positive numbers on the ophthalmoscope's lens disc to focus on near objects such as the patient's cornea and lens. Use the red, minus numbers to focus on distant objects such as the retina.

Aperture

Lens disc

Indicator of diopters

An opaque lens indicates cataracts. You may not be able to complete your examination.

Retinal structures

To examine the retina, start with the lens disc turned to zero. Rotate the lens disc to adjust for your refractive correction and the patient's refractive error. The first retinal structures you'll see are the blood vessels. Rotate the lens disc into the negative numbers to bring the blood vessels into focus.

Follow one of the vessels along its path toward the nose until you reach the optic disk. Examine arteriovenous crossings for localized constrictions in the retinal vessels, which might be a sign of hypertension.

Optic disk

The optic disk is a creamy pink to yellow-orange structure with clear borders and a round-to-oval shape; the physiologic cup is a small depression that occupies about one-third of the disk's diameter.

Retina

Completely scan the retina by following four blood vessels from the optic disk to different peripheral areas. The retina should have a uniform color and be free from scars and pigmentation.

Macula

Move the light laterally from the optic disk to locate the macula, the part of the eye most sensitive to light. It appears as a darker structure, free from blood vessels.

The fundus

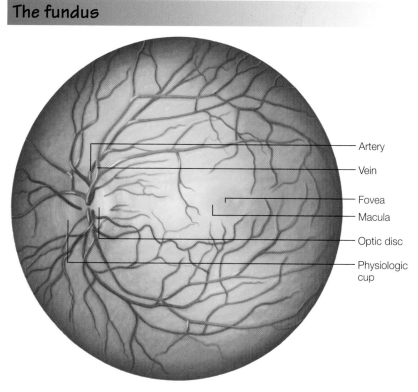

Artery
Vein
Fovea
Macula
Optic disc
Physiologic cup

Ears

External observation

Observe the ears for position and symmetry. The top of the ear should line up with the outer corner of the eye, and the ears should look symmetrical, with an angle of attachment of no more than 10 degrees.

Inspect the auricle for lesions, drainage, nodules, or redness. Pull the helix back and note if it's tender, which may indicate otitis externa. Inspect and palpate the mastoid area behind each auricle, noting tenderness, redness, or warmth.

Finally, inspect the opening of the ear canal, noting discharge, redness, odor, or the presence of nodules or cysts. Patients normally have varying amounts of hair and cerumen (earwax) in the ear canal.

> The top of the ear should line up with the outer corner of the eye and the ears should look symmetrical with an angle of attachment of no more than 10 degrees.

External ear (auricle)

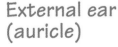

- Helix
- Anthelix
- Triangular fossa
- Crus
- External acoustic meatus
- Tragus
- Antitragus
- Lobule of auricle

Genes and the cerumen scene

The presence of cerumen in the ear canal doesn't indicate poor hygiene. In fact, the appearance and type of cerumen is genetically determined. There are two types of cerumen:

- dry cerumen — gray and flaky; mostly found in Asians and Native Americans (including Eskimos)
- wet cerumen — dark brown and moist; commonly found in Blacks and Whites.

best picture

Otoscopic examination

Positioning the patient

Ask the patient to sit with his back straight and head tilted away from you and toward the opposite shoulder. Straighten the ear canal by grasping the auricle and pulling it up and back.

Positioning the scope

Hold the otoscope handle between your thumb and fingers and brace your hand firmly against the patient's head. Doing so keeps you from hitting the canal with the speculum.

Inserting the speculum

Insert the speculum one-third its length gently down and forward into the ear canal. Be careful not to touch either side of the inner portion of the ear canal wall because this area is covered by a thin epithelial layer that's sensitive to pressure.

Viewing the structures

Once the otoscope is positioned properly, you should see the tympanic membrane, pars flaccida, and the bony structures, as shown. The tympanic membrane should be pearl gray, glistening, and transparent. Inspect the membrane for bulging, retraction, bleeding, lesions, and perforations.

The light reflex in the right ear should be between 4 and 6 o'clock; in the left ear it should be between 6 and 8 o'clock. Finally, look for the bony landmarks. The malleus will appear as a dense, white streak at 12 o'clock. The umbo is the inferior portion of the malleus.

Right eardrum

- Pars flaccida
- Short process of malleus
- Handle of malleus
- Umbo
- Light reflex

An elderly patient's tympanic membrane may appear cloudy.

best picture

Hearing acuity tests

Test the patient's hearing using Weber's test and the Rinne test. These tests assess conduction hearing loss, impaired sound transmission to the inner ear, sensorineural hearing loss, and impaired auditory nerve conduction or inner ear function.

Weber's test

In Weber's test, a tuning fork is used to evaluate bone conduction. The tuning fork should be tuned to the frequency of normal human speech, 512 cycles/second. To perform Weber's test:
- Strike the tuning fork lightly against your hand.
- Place the vibrating fork on the patient's forehead at the midline or on the top of his head.

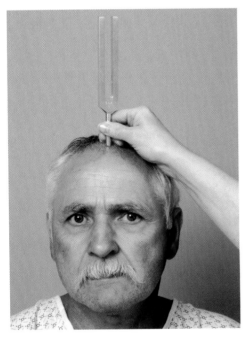

Results	Description
Normal	Patient hears tone equally well in both ears.
Right or left lateralization	Patient hears tone better in one ear.
Conductive hearing loss	Patient hears tone only in his impaired ear.
Sensorineural hearing loss	Patient hears tone only in his unaffected ear.

Rinne test

The Rinne test is used to compare air conduction (AC) of sound with bone conduction (BC) of sound. To perform this test:

- Strike the tuning fork against your hand.
- Place the vibrating fork over the patient's mastoid process.

Be sure to perform the Rinne test after you perform Weber's test.

- Ask the patient to tell you when the tone stops; note this time in seconds.

- Move the still-vibrating tuning fork to the ear's opening without touching the ear.

- Ask the patient to tell you when the tone stops; note this time in seconds.

Results	Description
Normal hearing	Patient hears AC tone twice as long as he hears BC tone (AC > BC).
Conductive hearing loss	Patient hears BC tone as long as or longer than he hears AC tone (BC ≥ AC).
Sensorineural hearing loss	Patient hears AC tone longer than he hears BC tone (AC > BC).

Eye abnormalities

Conjunctivitis

This condition is characterized by hyperemia of the conjunctiva with predominate redness in the eye periphery. It usually begins in one eye and rapidly spreads by contamination to the other eye. The patient experiences mild discomfort rather than severe pain. Vision isn't affected except for some blurring because of watery or mucopurulent eye discharge.

Hyperemia of the conjunctiva

Discharge and tearing

He can try to get the red out, but it won't work as long as I'm around.

Acute angle-closure glaucoma

Acute angle-closure glaucoma is characterized by a rapid onset of unilateral inflammation, severe eye pain and pressure, and photophobia. It also causes decreased vision, moderate pupil dilation, nonreactive pupillary response, and clouding of the cornea but no eye discharge. Ophthalmoscopic examination reveals changes in the retinal vessels and enlargement of the physiologic cup.

Disk changes associated with glaucoma

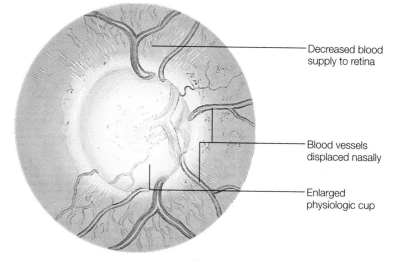

Decreased blood supply to retina

Blood vessels displaced nasally

Enlarged physiologic cup

outside the norm

Periorbital edema

Swelling around the eyes, or periorbital edema, may result from allergies, local inflammation, fluid-retaining disorders, or crying.

Ptosis

Ptosis, or a drooping upper eyelid, may be caused by an interruption in sympathetic innervation to the eyelid, muscle weakness, or damage to the oculomotor nerve.

Cataract

A common cause of vision loss, a cataract is an opacity of the lens or lens capsule of the eye that develops gradually.

Cornea (cut)

Lens with
■ protein aggregation
■ oxidative injury
■ increased pigmentation

Iris

Retina

Macular degeneration

Macular degeneration—atrophy or degeneration of the macular disk—is a cause of severe irreversible loss of central vision in people older than age 50. Age-related macular degeneration results from the formation of drusen or subretinal neovascular membrane changes in the macular region.

Retinal changes in macular degeneration

Macula

Drusen

Optic disk

Hardening and obstruction of retinal arteries

Keep an eye out for these eye abnormalities, too!

Decreased visual acuity

Decreased visual acuity—the inability to see clearly—commonly occurs with refractive errors. In nearsightedness, or *myopia*, vision at a distance is blurry. In farsightedness, or *hyperopia*, vision in close view is blurry.

Diplopia

Diplopia, or *double vision*, occurs when the extraocular muscles are misaligned.

Discharge

Discharge may occur in one or both eyes and may be scant or copious. The discharge may be purulent, frothy, mucoid, cheesy, serous, or clear or may have a stringy, white appearance. Eye discharge commonly results from inflammatory and infectious eye disorders such as conjunctivitis.

Pain

Eye pain may signal an emergency and requires immediate attention. Diseases causing eye pain include acute angle-closure glaucoma and blepharitis. Corneal damage caused by a foreign body or abrasions as well as trauma to the eye can also cause eye pain.

Vision loss

Disorders of any structure of the eye can result in vision loss. Types of vision loss include central vision loss, peripheral vision loss, or a blind spot in the middle of an area of normal vision (scotoma).

Visual halos

Increased intraocular pressure, which occurs in glaucoma, causes the patient to see halos and rainbows around bright lights.

Ear abnormalities

Earache

Earaches usually result from disorders of the external and middle ear and are associated with infection, hearing loss, and otorrhea.

Hearing loss

Several factors can interfere with the ear's ability to conduct sound waves. Cerumen, a foreign body, or a polyp may obstruct the ear canal. Otitis media may thicken the fluid in the middle ear, which interferes with the vibrations that transmit sound. Otosclerosis, a hardening of the bones in the middle ear, also interferes with the transmission of sound vibrations. Trauma can disrupt the middle ear's bony chain.

Otitis media

Otitis media, inflammation of the middle ear, results from disruption of eustachian tube patency. It can be suppurative or secretory, acute (as shown at right) or chronic.

Acute otitis media

■ Infected fluid in middle ear
■ Rapid onset and short duration

Otoscopic view

Complications of otitis media

Otitis media with effusion

■ Characterized by fluid in middle ear that may not cause symptoms

■ May be acute, subacute, or chronic

Cholesteatoma

■ Abnormal skin growth or epithelial cyst in middle ear that usually results from repeated ear infections

Perforation

■ Hole in tympanic membrane caused by chronic negative middle ear pressure, inflammation, or trauma

Able to label?

Identify the intra-ocular structures indicated on this illustration.

1. _____
2. _____
3. _____
4. _____

5. _____
6. _____

Show and tell

Describe the steps for performing the Rinne test, including those shown at right.

1. _____
2. _____
3. _____

4. _____
5. _____

Answers: Able to label? 1. Lens, 2. Cornea, 3. Pupil, 4. Iris, 5. Vitreous humor, 6. Optic nerve; Show and tell 1. Strike the tuning fork against your hand. 2. Place the vibrating fork over the patient's mastoid process. 3. Ask the patient to tell you when the tone stops; note this time in seconds. 4. Move the still-vibrating tuning fork to the ear's opening without touching the ear. 5. Ask the patient to tell you when the tone stops; note this time in seconds.

4

Nose, mouth, throat, and neck

I just "nose" that there's some good assessment advice in here.

Anatomy

Nose

The lower two-thirds of the external nose consists of flexible cartilage, and the upper one-third is rigid bone. Posteriorly, the internal nose merges with the pharynx, which is divided into the *nasopharynx*, *oropharynx*, and *laryngopharynx*. Anteriorly, it merges with the external nose.

More than just the sensory organ of smell, the nose also plays a key role in the respiratory system by filtering, warming, and humidifying inhaled air.

The internal and external nose are divided vertically by the nasal septum. Kiesselbach's area, the most common site of nosebleeds, is located in the anterior portion of the septum. Air entering the nose passes through the vestibule, which is lined with coarse hair that helps filter dust.

Nasopharyngeal structures

- Frontal sinus
- Sella turcica
- Sphenoid sinus
- Ethmoidal sinus
- Maxillary sinus
- Pharyngeal tonsil
- Eustachian tube opening
- Hard palate
- Soft palate
- Nasopharynx
- Palatine tonsil
- Tongue
- Oropharynx
- Laryngopharynx

Sinuses

Four pairs of paranasal sinuses open into the internal nose:
- maxillary sinuses, located on the cheeks below the eyes
- frontal sinuses, located above the eyebrows
- ethmoidal and sphenoidal sinuses, located behind the eyes and nose in the head.

   The sinuses serve as resonators for sound production and provide mucus. You'll be able to assess the maxillary and frontal sinuses, but the ethmoidal and sphenoidal sinuses aren't readily accessible.

Paranasal sinuses
Anterior view

- Frontal sinus
- Ethmoidal sinus
- Nasal cavity
- Middle nasal concha
- Middle nasal meatus
- Maxillary sinus
- Inferior nasal concha
- Inferior nasal meatus
- Nasal septum

Lateral view

Frontal sinus
Ethmoidal sinuses
- Posterior
- Middle
- Anterior
Sphenoidal sinus
Nasal cavity
Maxillary sinus
Middle nasal meatus
Inferior nasal meatus

Mouth and throat

The mouth is bounded by the lips, cheeks, palate, and tongue and contains the teeth. The throat, or pharynx, contains the hard and soft palates, the uvula, and the tonsils.

Structures of the mouth and throat

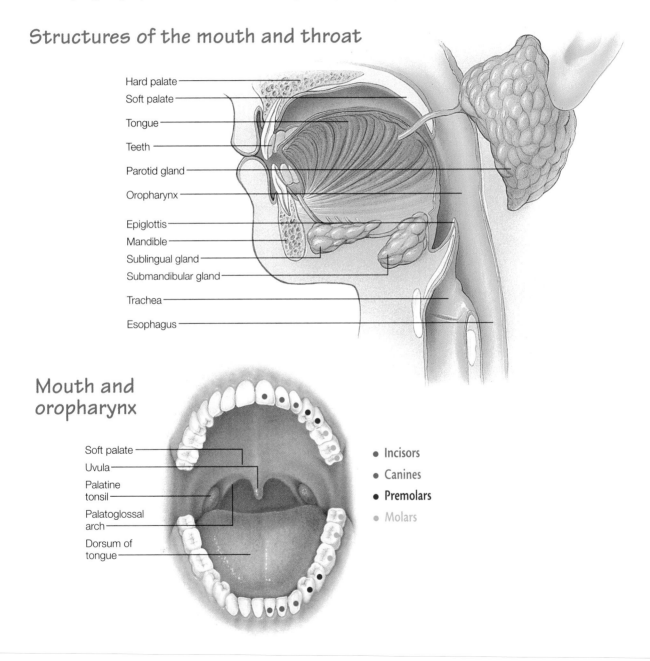

Hard palate
Soft palate
Tongue
Teeth
Parotid gland
Oropharynx
Epiglottis
Mandible
Sublingual gland
Submandibular gland
Trachea
Esophagus

Mouth and oropharynx

Soft palate
Uvula
Palatine tonsil
Palatoglossal arch
Dorsum of tongue

- Incisors
- Canines
- **Premolars**
- Molars

Neck

The neck is formed by the cervical vertebrae, the major neck and shoulder muscles, and their ligaments. Other important structures of the neck include the trachea, thyroid gland, and chains of lymph nodes.

The thyroid gland lies in the anterior neck, just below the larynx. Its two cone-shaped lobes are located on either side of the trachea and are connected by an isthmus below the cricoid cartilage, which gives the gland its butterfly shape.

Structures of the neck

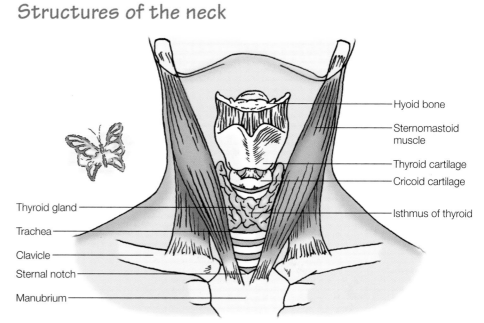

- Hyoid bone
- Sternomastoid muscle
- Thyroid cartilage
- Cricoid cartilage
- Isthmus of thyroid
- Thyroid gland
- Trachea
- Clavicle
- Sternal notch
- Manubrium

Lymph node locations

- Occipital
- Tonsillar
- Superficial cervical
- Anterior cervical
- Posterior cervical
- Supraclavicular
- Preauricular
- Postauricular
- Submandibular
- Submental

Assessment

Nose and sinuses

Inspecting the nose

Observe the patient's nose for position, symmetry, and color. Note variations, such as discoloration, swelling, or deformity. Variations in size and shape are largely caused by differences in cartilage and in the amount of fibroadipose tissue.

Observe for nasal discharge or flaring. If discharge is present, note the color, quantity, and consistency. If you notice flaring, observe for other signs of respiratory distress. Then inspect the nasal cavity.

Examine the nostrils by direct inspection using a nasal speculum, a penlight or small flashlight, or an otoscope with a short, wide-tip attachment.

best picture

Inspecting the nasal cavity

To inspect the nose, ask the patient to tilt his head back slightly, and then push up the tip of the nose and gently insert the otoscope. Use the light from the otoscope to illuminate the nasal cavities. Check for severe deviation or perforation of the nasal septum. Examine the vestibule and turbinates for redness, softness, swelling, and discharge.

> I'd need a colossal otoscope or nasal speculum to examine these nostrils!

Inspecting the nostrils

Have the patient sit in front of you with his head tilted back. Put on gloves and insert the tip of the closed nasal speculum into one nostril to the point where the blade widens. Slowly open the speculum as wide as possible without causing discomfort, as shown. Shine the flashlight in the nostril to illuminate the area.

Observe the color and patency of the nostril, and check for exudate. The mucosa should be moist, pink to light red, and free from lesions and polyps. After inspecting one nostril, close the speculum, remove it, and inspect the other nostril.

- Nasal septum
- Nasal airway
- Middle turbinate
- Middle meatus
- Inferior meatus
- Inferior turbinate

Palpating the nose

Palpate the patient's nose with your thumb and forefinger, assessing for pain, tenderness, swelling, and deformity.

Examining the sinuses

Begin by checking for swelling around the eyes, especially over the sinus area. Then palpate the sinuses, checking for tenderness.

If the patient complains of tenderness during sinus palpation, transilluminate the sinuses to see if they're filled with fluid or pus. Transillumination can also help reveal tumors and obstructions.

To perform transillumination, darken the room and have the patient close his eyes. Place a penlight under the eyebrow and direct the light upward to illuminate the frontal sinuses. Place the penlight on the patient's cheekbone just below the eye and ask the patient to open his mouth. A red glow inside the oral cavity indicates normal maxillary sinuses.

Remember, only the frontal and maxillary sinuses are accessible; you won't be able to palpate the ethmoidal and sphenoidal sinuses.

best picture

Palpating the maxillary sinuses

To palpate the maxillary sinuses, gently press your thumbs on each side of the nose just below the cheekbones.

Frontal sinuses

Maxillary sinuses

Mouth and throat

Inspect the patient's lips. Then put on gloves and palpate the lips for lumps or surface abnormalities.

Using a tongue blade and a bright light, inspect the mouth. Have the patient open his mouth; then place the tongue blade on top of his tongue. Observe the gingivae, or gums. Then inspect the teeth; note their number, condition, and whether any are missing or crowded. If the patient is wearing dentures, ask him to remove them so you can inspect the gums underneath. Next, inspect the tongue and oropharynx.

> The lateral borders of the tongue should be smooth and even-textured.

Inspecting the tongue

Ask the patient to raise the tip of her tongue and touch her palate directly behind her front teeth. Inspect the ventral surface of the tongue and the floor of the mouth. Next, wrap a piece of gauze around the tip of the tongue and move the tongue first to one side then the other to inspect the lateral borders.

Lips

The lips should be pink, moist, symmetrical, and without lesions. They may have a bluish hue or flecked pigmentation in dark-skinned patients.

Oral mucosa

The oral mucosa should be pink, smooth, moist, and free from lesions and unusual odors. Increased pigmentation may occur in dark-skinned patients.

Gingivae (gums)

The gums should be pink and moist, with clearly defined margins at each tooth. They shouldn't be retracted.

Inspecting the oropharynx

Inspect the patient's oropharynx by asking him to open his mouth while you shine the penlight on the uvula and palate. You may need to insert a tongue blade into the mouth and depress the tongue. Place the tongue blade slightly off center to avoid eliciting the gag reflex. Ask the patient to say "Ahhh." Observe for movement of the soft palate and uvula.

- Soft palate
- Uvula
- Tonsil
- Nasopharynx

Finally, palpate the lips, tongue, and oropharynx. Note lumps, lesions, ulcers, or edema of the lips or tongue. Assess the patient's gag reflex by gently touching the back of the pharynx with a cotton-tipped applicator or the tongue blade. Doing so should produce a bilateral response.

Tongue

The tongue should be midline, moist, pink, and free from lesions. It should have a smooth posterior surface and slightly rough anterior surface with small fissures. It should move easily in all directions and lie straight to the front at rest.

Oropharynx and uvula

These structures should be pink and moist, without inflammation or exudates.

Tonsils

The tonsils should be pink and without hypertrophy.

Neck

Inspection

Observe the patient's neck. It should be symmetrical, and the skin should be intact. Note any scars. No visible pulsations, masses, swelling, venous distention, or thyroid gland or lymph node enlargement should be present. Ask the patient to move his neck through the entire range of motion and to shrug his shoulders.

Palpation

Palpate the patient's neck using the finger pads of both hands. Assess the lymph nodes for size, shape, mobility, consistency, temperature, and tenderness, comparing nodes on one side with those on the other.

best picture

Palpating the lymph nodes

Using the finger pads of both hands, bilaterally palpate the chain of lymph nodes in the following sequence:

■ preauricular—in front of the ear
■ postauricular—behind the ear, superficial to the mastoid process
■ occipital—at the base of the skull
■ tonsillar—at the angle of the mandible
■ submandibular—between the angle and the tip of the mandible
■ submental—behind the tip of the mandible
■ superficial cervical—superficially along the sternomastoid muscle
■ posterior cervical—along the edge of the trapezius muscle
■ deep anterior cervical—deep under the sternomastoid muscle
■ supraclavicular—just above and behind the clavicle, in the angle formed by the clavicle and sternomastoid muscle.

memory board

When assessing the neck, remember to **SPEND** some time evaluating these findings:
Swelling
Pulsations
Enlargement (of thyroid gland or lymph node)
Neck masses
Distention.

Preauricular

Submandibular

Supraclavicular

Then palpate the trachea, which is normally located midline in the neck, and the thyroid.

Palpating the trachea

Place your finger along one side of the trachea. Assess the distance between the trachea's outer edge and the sternocleidomastoid muscle. Then assess the distance on the other side, and compare the two distances. They should be the same.

Palpating the thyroid

To palpate the thyroid, stand behind the patient and put your hands around his neck, with the fingers of both hands over the lower trachea. Ask him to swallow as you feel the thyroid isthmus. The isthmus should rise with swallowing because it lies across the trachea, just below the cricoid cartilage.

Displace the thyroid to the right and then to the left, palpating both lobes for enlargement, nodules, tenderness, or a gritty sensation. Lowering the patient's chin slightly and turning toward the side you're palpating helps relax the muscle and may facilitate assessment.

Palpating the thyroid

Normal thyroid on swallowing

Auscultation

Using light pressure on the bell of the stethoscope, listen over the carotid arteries. Ask the patient to hold his breath while you listen to prevent breath sounds from interfering with the sounds of circulation. Listen for bruits, which signal turbulent blood flow.

If you detect an enlarged thyroid gland during palpation, also auscultate the thyroid area with the bell. Check for a bruit or a soft rushing sound, which indicates a hypermetabolic state.

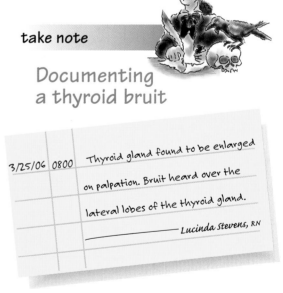

take note

Documenting a thyroid bruit

3/25/06 0800   Thyroid gland found to be enlarged on palpation. Bruit heard over the lateral lobes of the thyroid gland.

— Lucinda Stevens, RN

Nose abnormalities

outside the norm

Symptom synopsis: The nose

Symptom	Key facts	Possible causes
Epistaxis	▪ Refers to nosebleed	▪ Coagulation disorders ▪ Trauma ▪ Other hematologic disorders ▪ Renal disorders
Flaring	▪ Refers to dilation that occurs during inspiration ▪ Normal to some extent during quiet breathing but marked regular flaring is abnormal	▪ Respiratory distress
Stuffiness and discharge	▪ Refers to obstruction of the nasal mucous membranes accompanied by secretions	▪ Common cold ▪ Sinusitis ▪ Trauma ▪ Allergies ▪ Exposure to irritants ▪ Deviated septum

> Get to "nose" these common nasal problems.

Mouth abnormalities

outside the norm

Herpes simplex (type 1)

Herpes simplex, a recurrent viral infection, is caused by *human herpesvirus.* It's transmitted by oral and respiratory secretions, affects the mucous membranes, and produces cold sores and fever blisters. After a brief period of prodromal tingling and itching, the primary lesions erupt as vesicles on an erythematous base, eventually rupturing and leaving a painful ulcer, followed by a yellow crust. Vesicles may form on any part of the oral mucosa, especially the lips, tongue, and cheek.

Angioedema

Angioedema, commonly associated with urticaria, is usually caused by an allergic reaction. It presents subcutaneously or dermally and produces nonpitted swelling of subcutaneous tissue and deep, large wheals

usually on the lips, hands, feet, eyelids, or genitalia. These swellings don't itch but may burn or tingle.

Leukoplakia

Leukoplakia involves painless, white patches that may appear on the tongue or the mucous membranes of the mouth. It results from chronic irritation of the mucous membranes due to chronic tobacco use, poor-fitting dentures, or a rough tooth. The white patches are considered precancerous lesions. Biopsy determines whether the lesions are malignant.

Candidiasis

Candidiasis of the oropharyngeal mucosa causes cream-colored or white patches on the tongue, mouth, or pharynx. Most cases of this infection are caused by *Candida albicans*. Although these fungi are part of

the body's normal flora, they can cause infection when changes—such as an elevated blood glucose level in a patient with diabetes or immunosuppression in a patient with human immunodeficiency virus—allow for their sudden proliferation.

Throat abnormalities

Symptom synopsis: The throat

Symptom	Key facts	Possible causes
Dysphagia	▪ Refers to difficulty swallowing	▪ Esophageal disorders ▪ Oropharyngeal, respiratory, neurologic, or collagen disorders ▪ Certain toxins and treatments
Throat pain	▪ Commonly known as a *sore throat* ▪ Refers to discomfort in any part of the pharynx ▪ Ranges from a sensation of scratchiness to severe pain	▪ Infection such as pharyngitis or tonsillitis ▪ Trauma ▪ Allergies ▪ Cancer or a systemic disorder ▪ Surgery ▪ Endotracheal intubation ▪ Mouth breathing ▪ Alcohol consumption ▪ Inhaling smoke or chemicals such as ammonia ▪ Vocal strain

See if you can swallow this information about common throat-related symptoms.

Tonsillitis

Acute tonsillitis commonly begins with a mild to severe sore throat. Tonsillitis may also produce dysphagia, fever, swelling and tenderness of the lymph nodes, and redness in the throat. With exudative tonsillitis, a white exudate appears on the tonsils.

Pharyngitis

Pharyngitis is an acute or chronic inflammation of the pharynx that produces a sore throat and slight difficulty swallowing. It's usually caused by a virus, such as a rhinovirus, coronavirus, or adenovirus. It may also be caused by a bacterial infection, such as from group a beta-hemolytic streptococci.

Diphtheria

Diphtheria is an acute, highly contagious, toxin-mediated infection caused by *Corynebacterium diphtheriae*. It causes a sore throat with rasping cough and leads to airway obstruction. The throat appears red with a thick, gray membrane covering the back of the throat.

Neck abnormalities

Simple (nontoxic goiter)

A simple or nontoxic goiter involves thyroid gland enlargement that isn't caused by inflammation or a neoplasm. It's commonly classified as endemic or sporadic. Thyroid enlargement may range from a mildly enlarged gland to massive multinodular goiter.

I vant to assess your neck.

Graves' disease (toxic goiter)

Graves' disease is the most common form of thyrotoxicosis, a metabolic imbalance that results from thyroid hormone overproduction. The classic features of Graves' disease are an enlarged thyroid, nervousness, heat intolerance, weight loss despite increased appetite, sweating, frequent bowel movements, tremor, palpitations, and exophthalmos.

Toxic multinodular goiter

Common in the elderly, toxic multinodular goiter is a form of thyrotoxicosis that involves overproduction of thyroid hormone by one or more autonomously functioning nodules within a diffusely enlarged gland. Multiple thyroid nodules can be felt on palpation.

Able to label?

Identify the neck structures indicated on this illustration.

1. _____
2. _____
3. _____
4. _____

Matchmaker

Match the throat abnormalities shown here with the disorders that cause them.

1. _____

2. _____

3. _____

A. Tonsillitis

B. Pharyngitis

C. Diphtheria

5
Respiratory system

I do declare, this chapter is like a breath of fresh air.

Anatomy

The structures of the respiratory system (the airways, lungs, bony thorax, respiratory muscles, and central nervous system) work together to deliver oxygen to the bloodstream and remove excess carbon dioxide from the body.

Upper airways

The upper airways include the nasopharynx (nose), oropharynx (mouth), laryngopharynx, and larynx. These structures warm, filter, and humidify inhaled air.

Lower airways

The lower airways begin with the trachea, or windpipe, which extends from the cricoid cartilage to the carina. The trachea then divides into the right and left mainstem bronchi, which continue to divide all the way down to the alveoli, the gas-exchange units of the lungs.

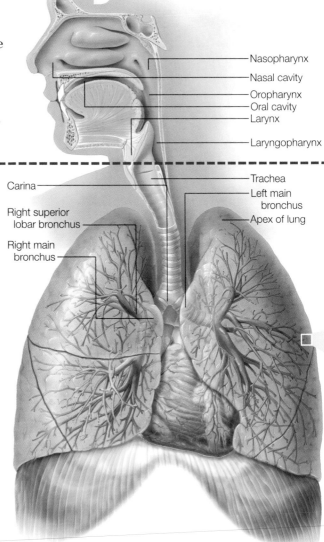

Upper airways

Lower airways

Nasopharynx
Nasal cavity
Oropharynx
Oral cavity
Larynx
Laryngopharynx

Carina
Right superior lobar bronchus
Right main bronchus

Trachea
Left main bronchus
Apex of lung

The larynx

The larynx houses the vocal cords. It's the transition point between the upper and lower airways. The epiglottis, a flap of tissue that closes over the top of the larynx when the patient swallows, protects the patient from aspirating food or fluid into the lower airways.

Anterior view

- Epiglottis
- Hyoid bone
- Thyrohyoid membrane
- Thyroid cartilage
- Oblique line
- Median cricothyroid ligament
- Inferior horn of thyroid cartilage
- Cricothyroid muscle (straight and oblique)
- Greater horn of hyoid bone
- Lesser horn of hyoid bone
- Median thyrohyoid ligament
- Lateral thyrohyoid ligament
- Superior thyroid notch
- Inferior thyroid notch
- Cricoid cartilage (arch)
- Tracheal cartilage
- Trachea

Lower airways

- Trachea
- Mainstem bronchi
- Lobar bronchi
- Secondary bronchi
- Tertiary bronchi
- Terminal bronchioles
- Respiratory bronchioles
- Alveolar ducts
- Alveoli

- Smooth muscle
- Respiratory bronchiole
- Alveolar duct
- Alveolar pore
- Terminal bronchiole
- Pulmonary vein
- Pulmonary artery
- Alveoli
- Capillary bed
- Alveolar sac

Lungs

The right lung has three lobes: upper, middle, and lower. The left lung is smaller and has only an upper and a lower lobe. The lungs share space in the thoracic cavity with the heart and great vessels, the trachea, the esophagus, and the bronchi. The space between the lungs is called the *mediastinum.*

Thorax

The bony thorax includes the clavicles, sternum, scapula, 12 sets of ribs, and 12 thoracic vertebrae.

Respiratory muscles

The diaphragm and the external inter-costal muscles are the primary muscles used in breathing. They contract when the patient inhales and relax when the patient exhales. Accessory inspiratory muscles include the trapezius, sterno-cleidomastoid, and scalenes, which combine to elevate the scapulae, clavicles, sternum, and upper ribs.

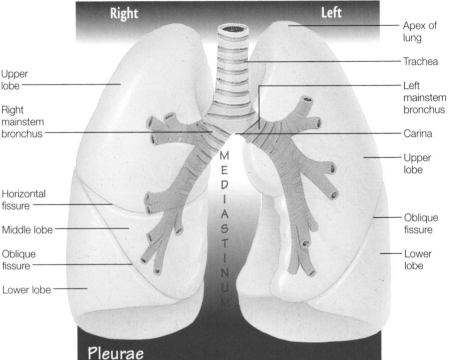

Right — Left

Upper lobe

Right mainstem bronchus

Horizontal fissure

Middle lobe

Oblique fissure

Lower lobe

MEDIASTINUM

Apex of lung

Trachea

Left mainstem bronchus

Carina

Upper lobe

Oblique fissure

Lower lobe

Pleurae

Each lung is wrapped in a lining called the *visceral pleura.* All areas of the thoracic cavity that come in contact with the lungs are lined with parietal pleura. A small amount of pleural fluid fills the area between the two layers of the pleura and allows the layers to slide smoothly over each other as the chest expands and contracts.

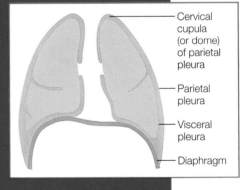

Cervical cupula (or dome) of parietal pleura

Parietal pleura

Visceral pleura

Diaphragm

The medulla's respiratory center initiates each breath by sending messages via the phrenic nerve to the primary respiratory muscles.

Assessment

Begin your respiratory assessment by first observing the patient's general appearance. Then use inspection, palpation, percussion, and auscultation to perform a physical examination. Examine the back of the chest first, comparing one side with the other. Then examine the front of the chest using the same sequence.

Inspecting the chest

Inspect for chest-wall symmetry. Note masses or scars that indicate trauma or surgery.

Respiratory assessment landmarks

These illustrations show the anterior and posterior landmarks of the respiratory system. You can use these landmarks to help describe the locations of your assessment findings.

Anterior view

- Suprasternal notch
- Manubrium
- Angle of Louis
- Right upper lobe
- Right middle lobe
- Right lower lobe
- Xiphoid process
- Clavicle
- First rib
- Left upper lobe
- Body of the sternum
- Left lower lobe

Landmark lines key

- Axillary line
- Midclavicular line
- Midsternal line
- Scapular line
- Vertebral line

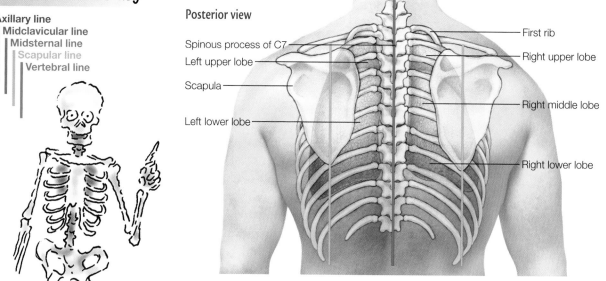

Posterior view

- Spinous process of C7
- Left upper lobe
- Scapula
- Left lower lobe
- First rib
- Right upper lobe
- Right middle lobe
- Right lower lobe

Respiratory rate and pattern

Count the number of breaths for a full minute. Adults normally breathe at a rate of 12 to 20 breaths/minute. An infant's breathing rate may reach 40 breaths/minute. The respiratory pattern should be even, coordinated, and regular, with occasional sighs.

Accessory muscle use

Observe the diaphragm and the intercostal muscles with breathing. Frequent use of accessory muscles may indicate a respiratory problem, particularly when the patient purses his lips and flares his nostrils when breathing.

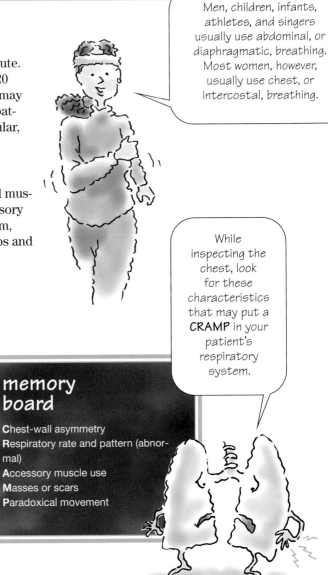

Men, children, infants, athletes, and singers usually use abdominal, or diaphragmatic, breathing. Most women, however, usually use chest, or intercostal, breathing.

While inspecting the chest, look for these characteristics that may put a **CRAMP** in your patient's respiratory system.

memory board

Chest-wall asymmetry
Respiratory rate and pattern (abnormal)
Accessory muscle use
Masses or scars
Paradoxical movement

Normal adult chest

Inspecting related structures

Inspect the skin, tongue, mouth, fingers, and nail beds. Patients with a bluish tint to their skin and mucous membranes are considered cyanotic. Clubbing of the fingers may signal long-term hypoxia.

Palpating the chest

The chest wall should feel smooth, warm, and dry. Gentle palpation shouldn't cause the patient pain. Pain may be caused by costochondritis, rib or vertebral fractures, or sore muscles as a result of protracted coughing. Crepitus, which feels like puffed-rice cereal crackling under the skin, indicates that air is leaking from the airways or lungs. Also palpate for tactile fremitus, palpable vibrations caused by the transmission of air through the bronchopulmonary system. Then evaluate chest-wall symmetry and expansion.

best picture

 Place your palm (or palms) lightly over the thorax. Palpate for tenderness, alignment, bulging, and retractions of the chest and intercostal spaces. Assess the patient for crepitus, especially around drainage sites. Repeat this procedure on the patient's back.

Use the pads of your fingers to palpate the front and back of the thorax. Pass your fingers over the ribs and any scars, lumps, lesions, or ulcerations. Note the skin temperature, turgor, and moisture. Also note tenderness or subcutaneous crepitus. The muscles should feel firm and smooth.

best picture

Checking for tactile fremitus

Ask the patient to fold his arms across his chest. This movement shifts the scapulae out of the way. Lightly place your open palms on both sides of the patient's back, as shown, without touching his back with his fingers. Ask the patient to repeat the phrase "ninety-nine" loud enough to produce palpable vibrations. Then palpate the front of the chest using the same hand positions.

What the results mean

Vibrations that feel more intense on one side than the other indicate tissue consolidation on that side. Less intense vibrations may indicate emphysema, pneumothorax, or pleural effusion. Faint or no vibrations in the upper posterior thorax may indicate bronchial obstruction or a fluid-filled pleural space.

Evaluating chest-wall symmetry and expansion

Place your hands on the front of the chest wall with your thumbs touching each other at the second intercostal space. As the patient inhales deeply, watch your thumbs. They should separate simultaneously and equally to a distance several centimeters away from the sternum. Repeat the measurement at the fifth intercostal space.

The same measurement may be made on the back of the chest near the tenth rib. The patient's chest may expand asymmetrically if he has pleural effusion, atelectasis, pneumonia, or pneumothorax.

Percussing the chest

Chest percussion reveals the boundaries of the lungs and helps to determine whether the lungs are filled with air or fluid or solid material.

best picture

■ Hyperextend the middle finger of your left hand if you're right-handed or the middle finger of your right hand if you're left-handed.
■ Place your hand firmly on the patient's chest.
■ Use the tip of the middle finger of your dominant hand to tap on the middle finger of your other hand just below the distal joint (as shown).

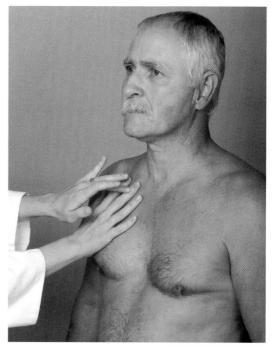

■ The movement should come from the wrist of your dominant hand, not your elbow or upper arm.
■ Follow the standard percussion sequence over the front and back chest walls.

Percussion sounds

Sound	Description	Clinical significance
Flat	Short, soft, high-pitched, extremely dull, as found over the thigh	Consolidation, as in atelectasis and extensive pleural effusion
Dull	Medium in intensity and pitch, moderate length, thudlike, as found over the liver	Solid area, as in lobar pneumonia
Resonant	Long, loud, low-pitched, hollow	Normal lung tissue; bronchitis
Hyperresonant	Very loud, lower-pitched, as found over the stomach	Hyperinflated lung, as in emphysema or pneumothorax
Tympanic	Loud, high-pitched, moderate length, musical, drumlike, as found over a puffed-out cheek	Air collection, as in a large pneumo-thorax

Diaphragmatic excursion

Percussion is also used to assess diaphragmatic excursion (the distance the diaphragm moves between inhalation and exhalation). Keep in mind that the diaphragm doesn't move as far in obese patients or patients with certain respiratory disorders.

best picture

Measuring diaphragm movement

■ Ask the patient to exhale.
■ Percuss the back on one side to locate the upper edge of the diaphragm, the point at which normal lung resonance changes to dullness.
■ Use a pen to mark the spot indicating the position of the diaphragm at full expiration on that side of the back.
■ Ask the patient to inhale as deeply as possible.
■ Percuss the back when the patient has breathed in fully until you locate the diaphragm. Use the pen to mark this spot as well.

■ Repeat on the opposite side of the back.
■ Use a ruler or tape measure to determine the distance between the pen marks. The distance, normally 1¼" to 2" (3 to 5 cm), should be equal on both the right and left sides.

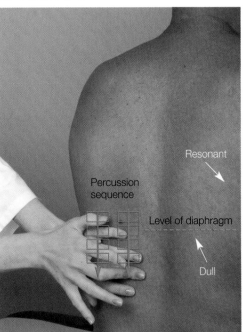

Resonant

Percussion sequence

Level of diaphragm

Dull

Auscultating the chest

As air moves through the bronchi, it creates sound waves that travel to the chest wall. The sounds produced by breathing change as air moves from larger airways to smaller airways. Sounds also change if they pass through fluid, mucus, or narrowed airways. Auscultation of these sounds helps you to determine the condition of the alveoli and surrounding pleura.

Classify each sound you hear according to its intensity, location, pitch, duration, and characteristic. Note whether the sound occurs when the patient inhales, exhales, or both.

Auscultation sequence

To distinguish between normal and adventitious breath sounds in the patient's lungs, press the diaphragm of the stethoscope firmly against the skin. Listen to a full inspiration and a full expiration at each site in the sequence shown. Remember to compare sound variations from one side to the other. Document adventitious sounds that you hear and include their locations.

The sequence used in percussion is also used for auscultation.

Anterior view

Posterior view

Listen to these auscultation tips

■ Have the patient breathe through his mouth; nose breathing alters the pitch of breath sounds.

■ If the patient has abundant chest hair, mat it down with a damp washcloth so the hair doesn't make sounds like crackles.

Assessing voice sounds

Check the patient for vocal fremitus—voice sounds resulting from chest vibrations that occur as the patient speaks. Abnormal transmission of voice sounds may occur over consolidated areas. The most common abnormal voice sounds are bronchophony, egophony, and whispered pectoriloquy.

Assessing vocal fremitus

- Ask the patient to repeat the words below while you listen.
- Auscultate over an area where you heard abnormally located bronchial breath sounds to check for abnormal voice sounds.

"ninety-nine"
Bronchophony
- Ask the patient to say, "ninety-nine."
- Over normal lung tissue, the words sound muffled.
- Over consolidated areas, the words sound unusually loud.

"E"
Egophony
- Ask the patient to say, "E."
- Over normal lung tissue, the sound is muffled.
- Over consolidated lung tissue, it will sound like the letter a.

"1, 2, 3"
Whispered pectoriloquy
- Ask the patient to whisper, "1, 2, 3."
- Over normal lung tissue, the numbers will be almost indistinguishable.
- Over consolidated lung tissue, the numbers will be loud and clear.

Locations of normal breath sounds

You'll hear four types of breath sounds over normal lungs. The type of sound you hear depends on where you listen. These illustrations show the normal locations of different types of breath sounds.

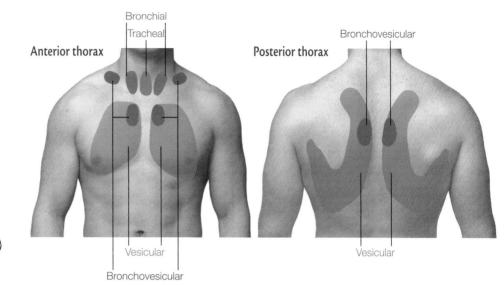

Anterior thorax

Bronchial
Tracheal

Posterior thorax

Bronchovesicular

Vesicular

Bronchovesicular

Vesicular

Qualities of normal breath sounds

Breath sound	Quality	Inspiration-expiration (I:E) ratio	Location	
Tracheal	Harsh, high-pitched	I = E	Above supraclavicular notch, over the trachea	
Bronchial	Loud, high-pitched	I < E	Just above clavicles on each side of the sternum, over the manubrium	
Bronchovesicular	Medium in loudness and pitch	I = E	Next to sternum, between scapulae	
Vesicular	Soft, low-pitched	I > E	Remainder of lungs	

Abnormal findings

Chest-wall abnormalities

Chest-wall abnormalities may be congenital or acquired. As you examine a patient for chest-wall abnormalities, keep in mind that a patient with a deformity of the chest wall might have completely normal lungs and that the lungs might be cramped within the chest. The patient might have a smaller-than-normal lung capacity and limited exercise tolerance, and he may more easily develop respiratory failure from a respiratory tract infection.

Paradoxical movement

Paradoxical (uneven) movement of the chest wall is abnormal. It can occur as a result of chest-wall injury, such as multiple rib fractures or blunt force trauma to the chest. With spontaneous breathing, paradoxical movement occurs on the injured chest side, which collapses during inspiration and expands during exhalation.

outside the norm

Chest deformities

Barrel chest

Increased anteroposterior diameter

Funnel chest
(pectus excavatum)

Depressed lower sternum

Pigeon chest
(pectus carinatum)

Anteriorly displaced sternum

Thoracic kyphoscoliosis

Raised shoulder and scapula, thoracic convexity, and flared interspaces

Abnormal respiratory patterns

Common abnormal respiratory patterns include tachypnea, bradypnea, apnea, hyperpnea, Kussmaul's respirations, Cheyne-Stokes respirations, and Biot's respirations.

outside the norm

Tachypnea

Shallow breathing with increased respiratory rate

Bradypnea

Decreased rate but regular breathing

Apnea

Absence of breathing; may be periodic

Hyperpnea

Deep, fast breathing

Kussmaul's respirations

Rapid, deep breathing without pauses; in adults, more than 20 breaths/minute; breathing usually sounds labored with deep breaths that resemble sighs

Cheyne-Stokes respirations

Breaths that gradually become faster and deeper than normal, then slower, and alternate with periods of apnea

Biot's respirations

Rapid, deep breathing with abrupt pauses between each breath; equal depth to each breath

Grading dyspnea

To assess dyspnea (shortness of breath) as objectively as possible, ask your patient to briefly describe how various activities affect his breathing. Then document his response using this grading system:

Grade 0	Not troubled by breathlessness except with strenuous exercise
Grade 1	Troubled by shortness of breath when hurrying on a level path or walking up a slight hill
Grade 2	Walks more slowly on a level path than people of the same age because of breathlessness or has to stop to breathe when walking on a level path at his own pace
Grade 3	Stops to breathe after walking approximately 100 yards (91 m) on a level path
Grade 4	Too breathless to leave the house or breathless when dressing or undressing

Abnormal breath sounds

If you hear a sound in an area other than where you would expect to hear it, consider the sound abnormal. For example, if you hear bronchial or bronchovesicular breath sounds in an area where you would normally hear vesicular breath sounds, then the alveoli and small bronchioles in that area might be filled with fluid or exudate, as occurs in pneumonia and atelectasis.

Adventitious sounds

Other breath sounds, called *adventitious sounds*, are abnormal no matter where you hear them in the lungs. These sounds, which are superimposed on normal breath sounds, include fine and coarse crackles, wheezes, rhonchi, stridor, and pleural friction rub.

Stridor is a loud, high-pitched crowing sound, usually heard without a stethoscope during auscultation. It's caused by upper airway obstruction.

Pleural friction rub is a low-pitched, grating, rubbing sound heard on inspiration and expiration. It's caused by pleural inflammation.

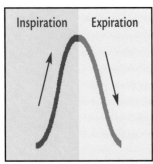

outside the norm

Discontinuous and continuous adventitious breath sounds

The characteristics of some discontinuous and continuous adventitious breath sounds are compared in the chart below. Note the timing of each sound during inspiration and expiration on the corresponding graphs.

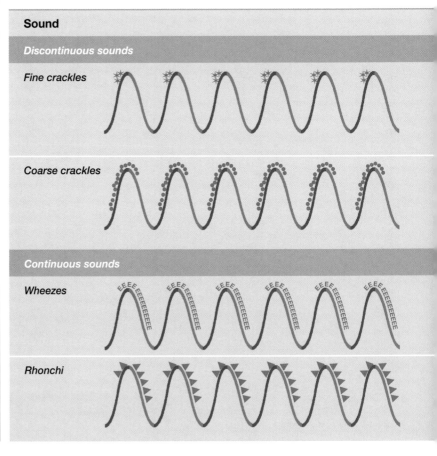

Sound
Discontinuous sounds
Fine crackles
Coarse crackles
Continuous sounds
Wheezes
Rhonchi

take note

Documenting
breath sounds

2/1/2006	1830	Pt. c/o shortness of breath and dizziness after walking from the bathroom. Skin cool and dry, color pale, lips and nail beds pink. Bilateral breath sounds with fine crackles in right lower and middle lobes. Respirations easy and regular without use of accessory muscles. BP 130/90, P 88/minute, RR 28/minute. Oxygen saturation 92% on room air. Dr. Ryan notified at 1820 and pt. placed on nasal O_2 at 4 L/minute and 12-lead ECG obtained. Wife at bedside. —————— Linda Martin, RN

Characteristics

- Intermittent
- Nonmusical
- Soft
- High-pitched
- Short, cracking, popping sounds
- Heard during inspiration

- Intermittent
- Nonmusical
- Loud
- Low-pitched
- Bubbling, gurgling sounds
- Heard during early inspiration and possibly during expiration

- Musical
- High-pitched
- Squeaky, whistling sounds
- Predominantly heard during expiration but may also occur during inspiration

- Musical
- Low-pitched
- Snoring, moaning sounds
- Heard during both inspiration and expiration but are more prominent during expiration

Auscultation findings for common disorders

Disorder	Auscultation findings
Asbestosis	▪ Bronchial breath sounds in both lung bases ▪ High-pitched crackles heard at the end of inspiration ▪ Pleural friction rub
Asthma	▪ Diminished breath sounds ▪ Musical, high-pitched expiratory polyphonic wheezes ▪ With status asthmaticus, loud and continuous random monophonic wheezes, along with prolonged expiration and possible silent chest if severe
Atelectasis	▪ High-pitched, hollow, tubular bronchial breath sounds, crackles, wheezes ▪ Fine, high-pitched, late inspiratory crackles ▪ Bronchophony, egophony, and whispered pectoriloquy when right upper lobe is affected
Bronchiectasis	▪ Profuse, low-pitched crackles heard during midinspiration

Keep in mind that the patient may not present with every abnormal breath sound listed for each disorder.

Disorder	Auscultation findings
Chronic obstructive pulmonary disease (COPD)	▪ Diminished, low-pitched breath sounds ▪ Sonorous or sibilant wheezes ▪ Inaudible bronchophony, egophony, and whispered pectoriloquy ▪ Prolonged expiration ▪ Fine inspiratory crackles
Pleural effusion	▪ Absent or diminished low-pitched breath sounds ▪ Occasionally loud bronchial breath sounds ▪ Normal breath sounds on contralateral side ▪ Bronchophony, egophony, and whispered pectoriloquy at upper border of pleural effusion
Pneumonia	▪ High-pitched, tubular bronchial breath sounds over affected area during inspiration and expiration ▪ Bronchophony, egophony, and whispered pectoriloquy ▪ Late inspiratory crackles not affected by coughing or position changes
Pneumothorax	▪ Absent or diminished low-pitched breath sounds ▪ Inaudible bronchophony, egophony, and whispered pectoriloquy ▪ Normal breath sounds on contralateral side
Upper airway obstruction	▪ Stridor ▪ Decreased or absent breath sounds ▪ Wheezing

Able to label?

Identify the respiratory structures indicated on this illustration.

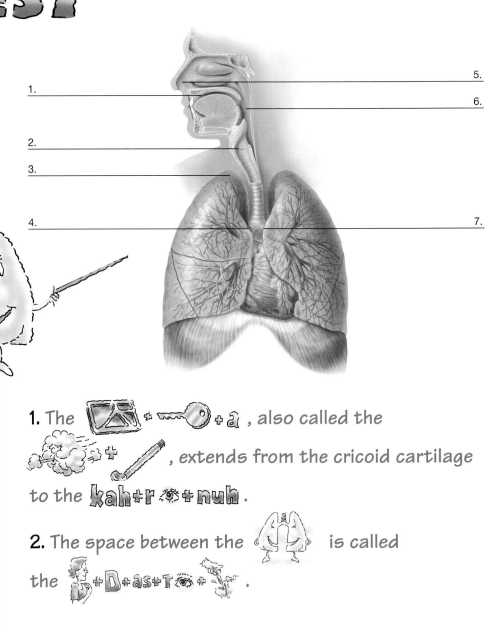

1. _____

2. _____

3. _____

4. _____

5. _____

6. _____

7. _____

Rebus riddle

Sound out each group of pictures and symbols to reveal terms that complete these two sentences about respiratory anatomy.

1. The [picture] + [key] + a , also called the [picture] + [picture] , extends from the cricoid cartilage to the **kah+r👁+nuh** .

2. The space between the [lungs] is called the [picture]+**D**+**as**+**r**👁+[fish] .

6 Cardiovascular system

Talk about action! The cardiovascular system is chock-full of it!

Anatomy of the heart

The heart is a hollow, muscular organ about the size of a closed fist. It's located between the lungs in the mediastinum, behind and to the left of the sternum. The heart spans the area from the second to the fifth intercostal space. Its right border aligns with the right border of the sternum. The left border aligns with the left midclavicular line.

The heart's location

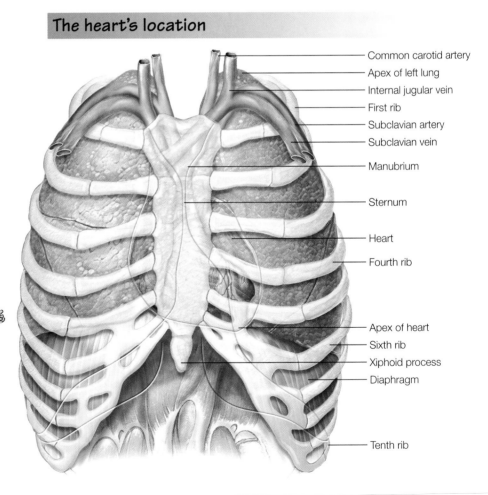

- Common carotid artery
- Apex of left lung
- Internal jugular vein
- First rib
- Subclavian artery
- Subclavian vein
- Manubrium
- Sternum
- Heart
- Fourth rib
- Apex of heart
- Sixth rib
- Xiphoid process
- Diaphragm
- Tenth rib

Keep in mind that the exact position of the heart may vary slightly with each patient.

Pericardium

The pericardium is a thin sac with an inner, or visceral, layer that forms the epicardium and an outer, or parietal, layer that protects the heart. The space between the two layers (the pericardial space) contains 10 to 30 ml of serous fluid, which prevents friction between the layers as the heart pumps.

Atria and ventricles

The heart has four chambers—two atria and two ventricles—separated by a cardiac septum. The upper atria have thin walls and serve as reservoirs for blood. They also boost the amount of blood moving into the lower ventricles, which fill primarily by gravity. The left ventricle pumps blood against a much higher pressure than the right ventricle, so its wall is three times thicker.

Layers of the heart wall

Fibrous pericardium

Parietal pericardium

Pericardial space

Epicardium

Myocardium

Endocardium

Structures of the heart

Superior vena cava

Aortic arch

Pulmonary artery

Left atrium

Right atrium

Left ventricle

Right ventricle

Anterior view

Vessels

Leading into and out of the heart are the great vessels: the inferior vena cava, the superior vena cava, the aorta, the pulmonary artery, and four pulmonary veins. Oxygenated blood travels through the pulmonary veins to the left atrium; it empties from the left atrium into the left ventricle, which pumps blood into the aorta. Deoxygenated venous blood returns to the right atrium through the superior vena cava, inferior vena cava, and coronary sinus.

Cardiac circulation

1 Deoxygenated venous blood returns to the right atrium through the superior vena cava, inferior vena cava, and coronary sinus.

2 Blood in the right atrium empties into the right ventricle, which contracts.

3 Blood is ejected through the pulmonic valve into the pulmonary artery, then travels to the lungs to be oxygenated.

4 From the lungs, blood travels to the left atrium through the pulmonary veins.

5 The left atrium empties the blood into the left ventricle, which then pumps the blood with each contraction through the aortic valve into the aorta and throughout the body.

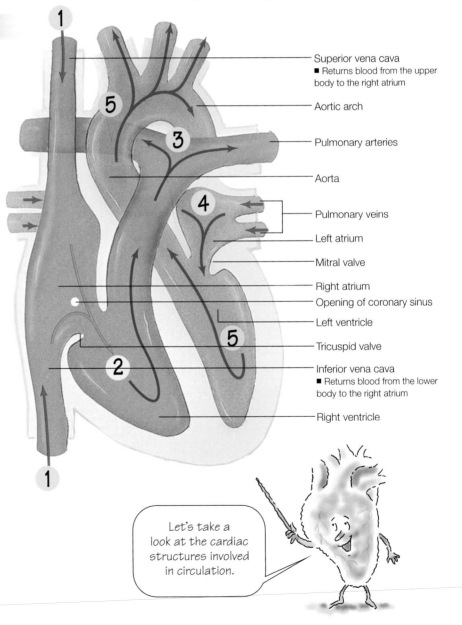

Superior vena cava
■ Returns blood from the upper body to the right atrium

Aortic arch

Pulmonary arteries

Aorta

Pulmonary veins

Left atrium

Mitral valve

Right atrium

Opening of coronary sinus

Left ventricle

Tricuspid valve

Inferior vena cava
■ Returns blood from the lower body to the right atrium

Right ventricle

Let's take a look at the cardiac structures involved in circulation.

Valves

Valves in the heart keep blood flowing in only one direction through the heart. Healthy valves open and close passively as pressure changes within the four heart chambers.

Locating the heart valves

Valves between the atria and ventricles are called *atrioventricular valves* and include the tricuspid valve on the right side of the heart and the mitral valve on the left. The pulmonic valve (between the right ventricle and pulmonary artery) and the aortic valve (between the left ventricle and the aorta) are called *semilunar valves*.

On the cusp

Each valve's leaflets, or cusps, are anchored to the heart wall by cords of fibrous tissue. Those cords, called *chordae tendineae,* are controlled by papillary muscles. The valves' cusps maintain tight closure. The tricuspid valve has three cusps. The mitral valve has two. The semilunar valves each have three cusps.

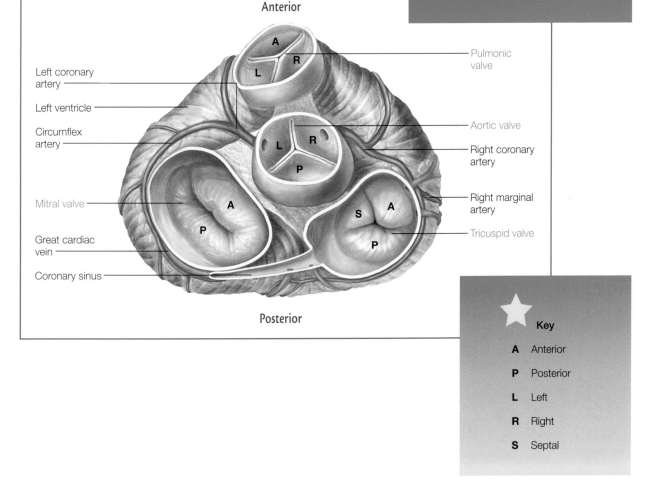

Anterior

Left coronary artery

Left ventricle

Circumflex artery

Mitral valve

Great cardiac vein

Coronary sinus

Pulmonic valve

Aortic valve

Right coronary artery

Right marginal artery

Tricuspid valve

Posterior

Key

A Anterior

P Posterior

L Left

R Right

S Septal

Physiology of the heart

Contractions of the heart occur in a rhythm—called the *cardiac cycle*—and are regulated by impulses that normally begin at the sinoatrial (SA) node.

Cardiac conduction

The heart's conduction system begins with the heart's pacemaker, the SA node. When an impulse leaves the SA node, it travels through the atria along Bachmann's bundle and the internodal pathways on its way to the atrioventricular (AV) node and the ventricles. After the impulse passes through the AV node, it travels to the ventricles, first down the bundle of His, then along the bundle branches and, finally, down the Purkinje fibers.

Bachmann's bundle

SA node

Internodal tract
- Posterior (Thorel's)
- Middle (Wenckebach's)
- Anterior

AV node

Bundle of His

Right bundle branch

Left bundle branch

Purkinje fibers

Anatomy of the vascular system

The vascular system delivers oxygen, nutrients, and other substances to the body's cells and removes the waste products of cellular metabolism. The peripheral vascular system consists of a network of about 60,000 miles of arteries, arterioles, capillaries, venules, and veins that's constantly filled with about 5 L of blood, which circulates to and from every functioning cell in the body.

Arteries

Arteries carry blood away from the heart. Nearly all arteries carry oxygen-rich blood from the heart throughout the rest of the body. The only exception is the pulmonary artery, which carries oxygen-depleted blood from the right ventricle to the lungs. Arteries are thick-walled because they transport blood under high pressure.

Capillaries

The exchange of fluid, nutrients, and metabolic wastes between blood and cells occurs in the capillaries. This exchange can occur because capillaries are thin-walled and highly permeable. Arterioles constrict and dilate to control blood flow to the capillaries. Venules gather blood from the capillaries.

Veins

Veins carry blood toward the heart. Most carry oxygen-depleted blood, with the exception of the pulmonary veins, which carry oxygenated blood from the lungs to the left atrium. Veins serve as a large reservoir for circulating blood. The wall of a vein is thinner and more pliable than the wall of an artery. Veins contain valves at periodic intervals to prevent blood from flowing backward.

A look at the cardiac cycle

The cardiac cycle consists of *systole,* the period when the heart contracts and sends blood on its outward journey, and *diastole,* the period when the heart relaxes and fills with blood.

Atrial systole

The atria contract, emptying blood into the ventricles. As pressure within the ventricles rises, the mitral and tricuspid valves snap shut, producing the first heart sound, S_1.

Ventricular systole

Shortly after atrial systole, the ventricles contract, ejecting blood from the heart to the lungs and the rest of the body. At the end of ventricular contraction, the aortic and pulmonic valves snap shut, producing the second heart sound, S_2.

Diastole

Atria and ventricles relax and blood refills each chamber.

Major veins and arteries of the vascular system

These illustrations show the major arteries and veins of the vascular system.

Major arteries

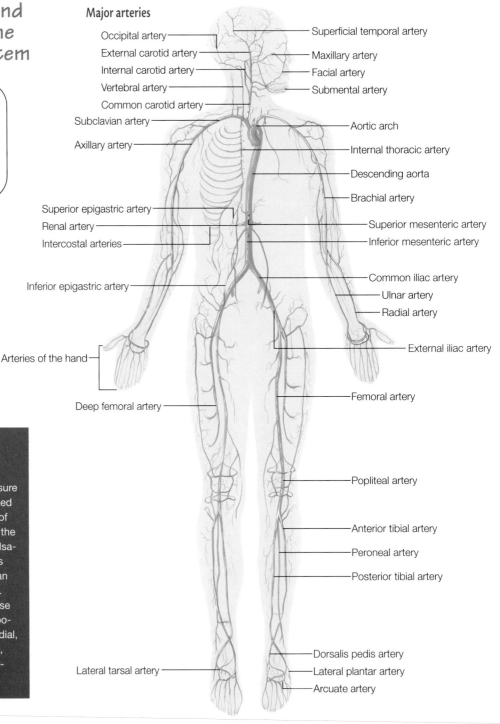

- Occipital artery
- External carotid artery
- Internal carotid artery
- Vertebral artery
- Common carotid artery
- Subclavian artery
- Axillary artery

- Superficial temporal artery
- Maxillary artery
- Facial artery
- Submental artery
- Aortic arch
- Internal thoracic artery
- Descending aorta
- Brachial artery

- Superior epigastric artery
- Renal artery
- Intercostal arteries
- Inferior epigastric artery

- Superior mesenteric artery
- Inferior mesenteric artery
- Common iliac artery
- Ulnar artery
- Radial artery
- External iliac artery

- Arteries of the hand
- Deep femoral artery

- Femoral artery
- Popliteal artery
- Anterior tibial artery
- Peroneal artery
- Posterior tibial artery

- Lateral tarsal artery

- Dorsalis pedis artery
- Lateral plantar artery
- Arcuate artery

Finger on the pulse

Arterial pulses are pressure waves of blood generated by the pumping action of the heart. All vessels in the arterial system have pulsations, but the pulsations can be felt only where an artery lies near the skin. You can palpate for these peripheral pulses: temporal, carotid, brachial, radial, ulnar, femoral, popliteal, posterior tibial, and dorsalis pedis.

Major veins

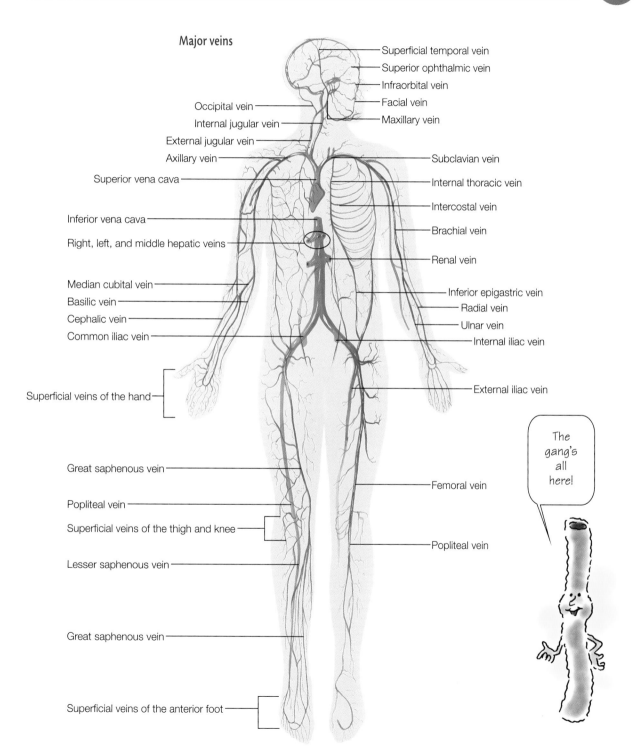

Superficial temporal vein
Superior ophthalmic vein
Infraorbital vein
Facial vein
Maxillary vein

Occipital vein
Internal jugular vein
External jugular vein
Axillary vein
Superior vena cava

Subclavian vein
Internal thoracic vein
Intercostal vein
Brachial vein

Inferior vena cava
Right, left, and middle hepatic veins

Renal vein

Median cubital vein
Basilic vein
Cephalic vein
Common iliac vein

Inferior epigastric vein
Radial vein
Ulnar vein
Internal iliac vein

Superficial veins of the hand

External iliac vein

Great saphenous vein

Femoral vein

Popliteal vein
Superficial veins of the thigh and knee
Lesser saphenous vein

Popliteal vein

Great saphenous vein

Superficial veins of the anterior foot

The gang's all here!

Assessment

As with assessment of other body systems, you'll inspect, palpate, percuss, and auscultate during your assessment of the cardiovascular system.

Assessing general appearance

First, take a moment to assess the patient's general appearance. Is he overly thin? Obese? Alert? Anxious? Note skin color, temperature, turgor, and texture. Are his fingers clubbed? (Clubbing is a sign of chronic hypoxia caused by a lengthy cardiovascular or respiratory disorder.) If the patient is dark-skinned, inspect his mucous membranes for pallor.

Assessing the neck vessels

Inspection

Inspect the vessels in the patient's neck. The carotid artery should appear to have a brisk, localized pulsation. The internal jugular vein has a softer, undulating pulsation. Unlike the pulsation of the carotid artery, pulsation of the internal jugular vein changes in response to position and breathing. The vein normally protrudes when the patient is lying down and lies flat when he stands.

> Inspecting the neck vessels can provide information about blood volume and pressure in the right side of the heart.

best picture

Evaluating jugular vein distention

■ With the patient in a supine position, position him so that you can visualize jugular vein pulsations reflected from the right atrium.

■ Elevate the head of the bed 45 to 90 degrees.

■ Locate the angle of Louis (sternal notch). To do so, palpate the clavicles where they join the sternum (the suprasternal notch). Place your first two fingers on the suprasternal notch. Then, without lifting them from the skin, slide them down the sternum until you feel a bony protuberance—this is the angle of Louis.

■ Find the internal jugular vein. (It indicates venous pressure more reliably than the external jugular vein.)

■ Shine a flashlight across the patient's neck to create shadows that highlight his venous pulse. Be sure to distinguish jugular vein pulsations from carotid artery pulsations. You can do this by palpating the vessel: Arterial pulsations continue, whereas venous pulsations disappear with light finger pressure. Also, venous pulsations increase or decrease with changes in body position; arterial pulsations remain constant.

■ Locate the highest point along the vein where you can see pulsations.

■ Using a centimeter ruler, measure the distance between the high point and the sternal notch. Record this finding as well as the angle at which the patient was lying. A finding greater than 1¼" to 1½" (3 to 4 cm) above the sternal notch, with the head of the bed at a 45-degree angle, indicates jugular vein distention.

Palpation

To palpate the carotid artery, lightly place your fingers just medial to the trachea and below the angle of the jaw. The pulse should be regular in rhythm and have equal strength in the right and left carotid arteries. You shouldn't be able to detect any palpable vibrations, known as *thrills*. Don't palpate both carotid arteries at the same time or press too firmly. If you do, the patient may faint or become bradycardic.

Auscultation

Normally, you should hear no vascular sounds over the carotid arteries upon auscultation. If you detect a blowing, swishing sound, this is a bruit that results from turbulent blood flow. A bruit can occur in patients with arteriosclerotic plaque formation.

best picture

Auscultating the carotid artery

Lightly place the bell of the stethoscope over the carotid artery, first on one side of the trachea, then on the other. Ask the patient to hold his breath if he can while you auscultate the artery. Doing so will help eliminate respiratory sounds that may interfere with your findings.

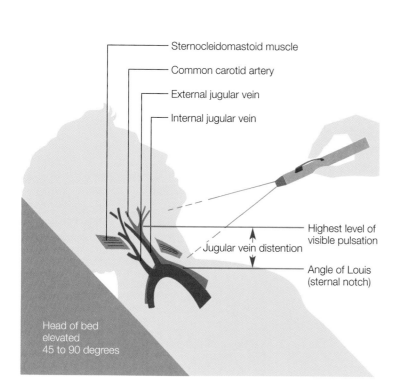

- Sternocleidomastoid muscle
- Common carotid artery
- External jugular vein
- Internal jugular vein
- Highest level of visible pulsation
- Jugular vein distention
- Angle of Louis (sternal notch)

Head of bed elevated 45 to 90 degrees

Assessing the heart

Inspection

Inspect the chest. Note landmarks you can use to describe your findings as well as structures underlying the chest wall. Look for pulsations, symmetry of movement, retractions, or heaves (strong outward thrusts of the chest wall that occur during systole).

Note the location of the apical impulse. This is also usually the point of maximal impulse and should be located in the fifth intercostal space at or just medial to the left midclavicular line. You'll notice it more easily in children and in patients with thin chest walls. To find the apical impulse in a woman with large breasts, displace the breasts during the examination.

Cardiovascular landmarks

Anterior thorax

Lateral thorax

- Sternoclavicular area
- Suprasternal notch
- Aortic area
- Pulmonic area
- Intercostal space
- Tricuspid area
- Mitral area
- Xiphoid process
- Epigastric area

Use these landmarks when describing your assessment findings.

Landmark lines key

- Axillary line (anterior)
- Axillary line (posterior)
- Midaxillary line
- Midclavicular line
- Midsternal line

Palpation

Maintain a gentle touch when you palpate so that you won't obscure pulsations or similar findings. Follow a systematic palpation sequence covering the sternoclavicular, aortic, pulmonic, tricuspid, and epigastric areas.

best picture

Palpating the apical impulse

To find the apical impulse, use the ball of your hand, then your fingertips, to palpate over the precordium. Note heaves or thrills, fine vibrations that feel like the purring of a cat.

Percussion

Percuss at the anterior axillary line and continue toward the sternum along the fifth intercostal space. The sound changes from resonance to dullness over the left border of the heart, normally at the midclavicular line. The right border of the heart is usually aligned with the sternum and can't be percussed.

Although percussing the heart isn't as useful as other methods of assessment, this technique may help you locate cardiac borders.

Auscultation

Use a zigzag pattern over the precordium. Be sure to listen over the entire precordium, not just over the valves. Note the heart rate and rhythm. Identify the first and second heart sounds (S_1 and S_2), then listen for adventitious sounds, such as third and fourth heart sounds (S_3 and S_4), murmurs, and pericardial friction rubs (scratchy, rubbing sounds).

best picture

Positioning the patient for auscultation

Auscultate for heart sounds with the patient in three positions: lying in a supine position with the head of the bed raised 30 to 45 degrees, lying on his left side, and sitting up.

For the supine position, have the patient lie on his back with the head of the bed elevated 30 to 45 degrees. Begin auscultation at the aortic area. Listen over all heart valve sites and the entire precordium. Use the diaphragm of the stethoscope to listen as you go in one direction, and use the bell as you come back in the other direction.

If heart sounds are faint or if you hear abnormal sounds, try listening to them with the patient lying on his left side (left lateral recumbent position) or seated and leaning forward.

Left lateral recumbent

The left lateral recumbent position is best suited for hearing low-pitched sounds, such as mitral valve murmurs and extra heart sounds. To hear these sounds, place the bell of the stethoscope over the apical area, as shown.

Leaning forward

To auscultate for high-pitched heart sounds related to semilunar valve problems, such as aortic and pulmonic valve murmurs, lean the patient forward. Place the diaphragm of the stethoscope over the aortic and pulmonic areas in the right and left second intercostal spaces, as shown.

Auscultating for heart sounds

1 Begin auscultating over the **aortic area,** placing the stethoscope over the second intercostal space, along the right sternal border.

2 Then move to the **pulmonic area,** located at the second intercostal space, at the left sternal border.

3 Next, assess the **tricuspid area,** which lies over the fourth and fifth intercostal spaces, along the left sternal border.

4 Finally, listen over the **mitral area,** located at the fifth intercostal space, near the midclavicular line.

You can learn a great deal about the heart by auscultating for heart sounds.

Follow the site path

■ In the **aortic area,** blood moves from the left ventricle during systole, crossing the aortic valve and flowing through the aortic arch.

■ In the **pulmonic area,** blood ejected from the right ventricle during systole crosses the pulmonic valve and flows through the main pulmonary artery.

■ In the **tricuspid area,** sounds reflect movement from the right atrium across the tricuspid valve, filling the right ventricle during diastole.

■ In the **mitral area,** also called the *apical area,* sounds represent blood flow across the mitral valve and left ventricular filling during diastole.

Heart sounds

Systole is the period of ventricular contraction. As pressure in the ventricles increases, the mitral and tricuspid valves snap closed. This closure produces the first heart sound, S_1. At the end of ventricular contraction, the aortic and pulmonic valves snap shut. This produces the second heart sound, S_2.

Always identify S_1 and S_2, then listen for adventitious sounds, such as third and fourth heart sounds (S_3 and S_4). Also listen for murmurs, which sound like vibrating, blowing, or rumbling sounds.

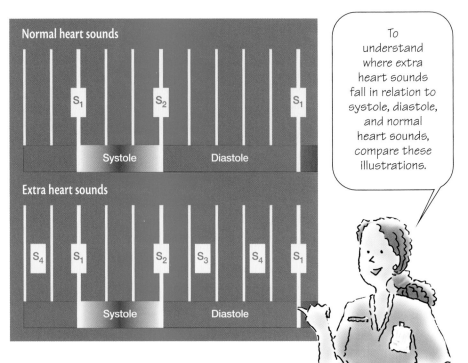

Normal heart sounds

S_1 S_2 S_1

Systole   Diastole

Extra heart sounds

S_4 S_1 S_2 S_3 S_4 S_1

Systole   Diastole

To understand where extra heart sounds fall in relation to systole, diastole, and normal heart sounds, compare these illustrations.

Auscultation tips

■ Concentrate as you listen for each sound.
■ Avoid auscultating through clothing or wound dressings because these items can block sound.
■ Avoid picking up extraneous sounds by keeping the stethoscope tubing off the patient's body and other surfaces.
■ Until you become proficient at auscultation, explain to the patient that listening to his chest for a long period doesn't mean that anything is wrong.
■ Ask the patient to breathe normally and to hold his breath periodically to enhance sounds that may be difficult to hear.

Hearing pericardial friction rubs

■ Have the patient lean forward because this position will bring the heart closer to the chest wall. If the patient can't tolerate leaning forward, position him sitting upright.
■ Ask the patient to exhale, then listen with the diaphragm of the stethoscope over the third intercostal space on the left side of the chest.
■ If you suspect a rub but have trouble hearing one, ask the patient to hold his breath.
■ A friction rub may be heard during atrial systole, ventricular systole, or ventricular diastole. As a result, the sounds produced by the rub may coincide with the first or second heart sound.
■ To differentiate a pericardial friction rub from a pleural friction rub, ask the patient to hold his breath. The sound from a pericardial friction rub persists, but the sound from a pleural friction rub ceases.

Assessing the vascular system

Inspection

Start by making general observations. Are the arms equal in size? Are the legs symmetrical? Then note skin color, body hair distribution, and lesions, scars, clubbing, and edema of the extremities. If the patient is confined to bed, check the sacrum for swelling. Examine the fingernails and toenails for abnormalities.

Palpation

First, assess skin temperature, texture, and turgor. Then assess capillary refill in the nail beds on the fingers and toes. Refill time should be no more than 3 seconds, or long enough to say "capillary refill." Palpate the patient's arms and legs for temperature and edema. Then palpate arterial pulses.

best picture

Palpating arterial pulses

Palpate for arterial pulses by gently pressing with the pads of your index and middle fingers. Start at the top of the patient's body at the temporal artery and work your way down. Palpate for the pulse on each side, comparing pulse volume and symmetry. All pulses should be regular in rhythm and equal in strength.

Carotid pulse

Lightly place your fingers just lateral to the trachea and below the jaw angle. Never palpate both carotid arteries at the same time.

Brachial pulse

Position your fingers medial to the biceps tendon.

Radial pulse

Apply gentle pressure to the medial and ventral side of the wrist, just below the base of the thumb.

Femoral pulse

Press relatively hard at a point inferior to the inguinal ligament. For an obese patient, palpate in the crease of the groin, halfway between the pubic bone and the hip bone.

(continued)

Popliteal pulse

Press firmly in the popliteal fossa at the back of the knee.

Posterior tibial pulse

Apply pressure behind and slightly below the malleolus of the ankle.

Dorsalis pedis pulse

Place your fingers on the medial dorsum of the foot while the patient points his toes down. The pulse is difficult to palpate here and may seem to be absent in healthy patients.

Grading pulses

∘ Pulses are graded on a four-point scale.

4+ = bounding

3+ = increased

2+ = normal

1+ = weak

0 = absent

Auscultation

Using the bell of the stethoscope, follow the palpation sequence and auscultate over each artery. Assess the upper abdomen for abnormal pulsations, which could indicate the presence of an abdominal aortic aneurysm. Finally, auscultate for the femoral and popliteal pulses, checking for a bruit or other abnormal sounds.

Abnormal findings

Skin and hair abnormalities

Warm skin may indicate conditions causing fever or increased cardiac output. Absence of body hair on the arms or legs may indicate diminished arterial blood flow to these areas. Cyanosis, pallor, or cool skin may indicate poor cardiac output and tissue perfusion.

outside the norm

Cyanosis and pallor

Cyanosis and pallor may indicate poor cardiac output and tissue perfusion.

Cyanosis

Pallor

Arterial and venous insufficiency

Arterial insufficiency

In a patient with arterial insufficiency, pulses may be decreased or absent. The skin is cool, pale, and shiny, hair loss occurs in the area, and the patient may have pain in the legs and feet. Ulcerations typically occur in the area around the toes, and the foot usually turns deep red when dependent. Nails may be thick and ridged.

Hair loss
Pale, shiny skin
Redness
Ulcer
Thick, ridged nails

Chronic venous insufficiency

In a patient with chronic venous insufficiency, ulcerations develop around the ankle. Pulses are present but may be difficult to find because of edema. The foot may become cyanotic when dependent.

Pitting edema
Brown pigment
Ulcer

Edema

Swelling, or edema, may indicate heart failure or venous insufficiency. Right-sided heart failure may cause swelling in the lower legs. Edema may also result from varicosities or thrombophlebitis.

outside the norm

Edema

Edema may be pitting or nonpitting. To differentiate between the two, press your finger against a swollen area for 5 seconds, then quickly remove it.

Pitting edema

With pitting edema, pressure forces fluid into the underlying tissues, causing an indentation that slowly fills. To determine the severity of pitting edema, estimate the indentation's depth in centimeters: 1+, 2+, 3+, or 4+.

Nonpitting edema

With nonpitting edema, pressure leaves no indentation because fluid has coagulated in the tissues. Typically, the skin feels unusually tight and firm.

Abnormal pulsations

A weak arterial pulse may indicate decreased cardiac output or increased peripheral vascular resistance; both point to arterial atherosclerotic disease. Strong or bounding pulsations usually occur in a patient with a condition that causes increased cardiac output, such as hypertension, hypoxia, anemia, exercise, or anxiety. A thrill usually suggests a valvular dysfunction.

Abnormal pulsation	What causes it
Displaced apical impulse	▪ Heart failure ▪ Hypertension
Forced apical impulse	▪ Increased cardiac output
Aortic, pulmonic, or tricuspid pulsation	▪ Valvular disease ▪ Heart chamber enlargement ▪ Aortic aneurysm (aortic pulsation only)
Epigastric pulsation	▪ Heart failure ▪ Aortic aneurysm
Sternoclavicular pulsation	▪ Aortic aneurysm
Slight left and right sternal pulsations	▪ Anemia ▪ Anxiety ▪ Increased cardiac output ▪ Thin chest wall
Sternal border heave	▪ Right ventricular hypertrophy ▪ Ventricular aneurysm

Abnormal pulses

These waveforms illustrate abnormal arterial pulses.

Weak pulse

A weak pulse has a decreased amplitude with a slower up-stroke and downstroke. Possible causes of a weak pulse include increased peripheral vascular resistance, as occurs in cold weather or with severe heart failure, and decreased stroke volume, as occurs with hypovolemia or aortic stenosis.

Bounding pulse

A bounding pulse has a sharp upstroke and downstroke with a pointed peak. The amplitude is elevated. Possible causes of a bounding pulse include increased stroke volume, as with aortic insufficiency, or stiffness of arterial walls, as with aging.

Pulsus alternans

Pulsus alternans has a regular, alternating pattern of a weak and a strong pulse. This pulse is associated with left-sided heart failure.

Pulsus bigeminus

Pulsus bigeminus is similar to pulsus alternans but occurs at irregular intervals. This pulse is caused by premature atrial or ventricular beats.

Pulsus paradoxus

Pulsus paradoxus has increases and decreases in amplitude associated with the respiratory cycle. Marked decreases occur when the patient inhales. Pulsus paradoxus is associated with pericardial tamponade, advanced heart failure, and constrictive pericarditis.

Pulsus biferiens

Pulsus biferiens shows an initial upstroke, a subsequent downstroke, then another upstroke during systole. Pulsus biferiens is caused by aortic stenosis and aortic insufficiency.

Abnormal heart sounds

Third heart sound

S_3 is a normal finding in children and young adults; however, an abnormal S_3 is commonly heard in patients with high cardiac output. Called *ventricular gallop* when it occurs in adults, S_3 may be a cardinal sign of heart failure.

Often compared to the y sound in "Ken-tuck-y," S_3 is low-pitched and occurs when the ventricles fill rapidly. It follows S_2 in early ventricular diastole. In addition to heart failure, S_3 may also be associated with conditions such as pulmonary edema, atrial septal defect, acute myocardial infarction (MI), and the last trimester of pregnancy.

S_3 is best heard at the apex when the patient is lying on his left side.

Fourth heart sound

S_4 is an abnormal sound called an *atrial gallop* that's heard over the tricuspid or mitral areas when the patient is on his left side. It indicates increased resistance to ventricular filling. You may hear S_4 in elderly patients or in those with hypertension, aortic stenosis, or a history of MI. S_4, commonly described as sounding like "Ten-nes-see," occurs just before S_1, after atrial contraction.

Pericardial friction rub

When inflamed pericardial surfaces rub together, they produce a characteristic high-pitched friction noise of grating or scratchy quality known as *pericardial friction rub*. A classic sign of inflammation of the pericardium (pericarditis), a pericardial friction rub may result from a viral or bacterial infection, radiation therapy to the chest, or cardiac trauma.

outside the norm

Abnormal heart sounds

Whenever auscultation reveals an abnormal heart sound, try to identify the sound and its timing in the cardiac cycle. Knowing those characteristics can help you identify the possible cause for the sound. Use this chart to put all that information together.

Abnormal heart sound
Accentuated S_1
Diminished S_1
Split S_1 (mitral and tricuspid components to the S_1 sound)
Accentuated S_2
Diminished or inaudible S_2
Persistent S_2 split (aortic and pulmonic components to the S_2 sound)
Reversed or paradoxical S_2 split that appears during exhalation and disappears during inspiration
S_3 (ventricular gallop)
S_4 (atrial or presystolic gallop)
Pericardial friction rub (grating or leathery sound at the left sternal border; usually muffled, high-pitched, and transient)

take note

Documenting heart sounds

Timing	Possible causes
Beginning of systole	Mitral stenosis or fever
Beginning of systole	Mitral insufficiency, heart block, or severe mitral insufficiency with a calcified, immobile valve
Beginning of systole	Right bundle-branch block (BBB) or premature ventricular contractions
End of systole	Pulmonary or systemic hypertension
End of systole	Aortic or pulmonic stenosis
End of systole	Delayed closure of the pulmonic valve, usually from overfilling of the right ventricle, causing prolonged systolic ejection time
End of systole	Delayed ventricular stimulation, left BBB, or prolonged left ventricular ejection time
Early diastole	Overdistention of the ventricles during the rapid-filling segment of diastole or mitral insufficiency or ventricular failure (normal in children and young adults)
Late diastole	Pulmonic stenosis, hypertension, coronary artery disease, aortic stenosis, or forceful atrial contraction due to resistance to ventricular filling late in diastole (resulting from left ventricular hypertrophy)
Throughout systole and diastole	Pericardial inflammation

| 4/3/2006 | 1530 | Pt. alert and oriented to time, place, and person. Skin warm and dry; lips and nail beds pink. Reports SOB with ambulation to the bathroom. Denies SOB at rest. Denies chest pain. Has occasional dry cough. Bilateral breath sounds with scattered bibasilar crackles. S_3 sound heard on auscultation, no JVD, 2+ pitting edema both ankles. Nasal O_2 at 2 L/minute. Call placed to Dr. Anderson's office at 1520. |
| | | —— Russ Wallace, RN |

Murmurs

If you identify a heart murmur, listen closely to determine its timing in the cardiac cycle. Then determine its other characteristics: quality (blowing, musical, harsh, or rumbling), pitch (medium, high, or low), and location (where the murmur sounds the loudest). Use a standard, six-level grading scale to describe the intensity (loudness) of the murmur.

outside the norm

Heart murmurs

Heart murmurs are described according to their timing, quality and pitch, and location. This chart outlines the various types of murmurs and their possible causes.

Timing	Quality and pitch	Location	Possible causes
Midsystolic (systolic ejection)	Harsh, rough with medium to high pitch	Pulmonic	Pulmonic stenosis
	Harsh, rough with medium to high pitch	Aortic and suprasternal notch	Aortic stenosis
Holosystolic (pansystolic)	Harsh with high pitch	Tricuspid	Ventricular septal defect
	Blowing with high pitch	Mitral, lower left sternal border	Mitral insufficiency
	Blowing with high pitch	Tricuspid	Tricuspid insufficiency
Early diastolic	Blowing with high pitch	Midleft sternal edge (not aortic area)	Aortic insufficiency
	Blowing with high pitch	Pulmonic	Pulmonic insufficiency
Mid-diastolic to late diastolic	Rumbling with low pitch	Apex	Mitral stenosis
	Rumbling with low pitch	Tricuspid, lower right sternal border	Tricuspid stenosis

Murmur grading

Grade 1—barely audible, even to the trained ear

Grade 2—clearly audible

Grade 3—moderately loud

Grade 4—loud with palpable thrill

Grade 5—very loud with a palpable thrill; can be heard when the stethoscope has only partial contact with the chest

Grade 6—extremely loud with a palpable thrill; can be heard with the stethoscope lifted just off the chest wall

Murmur configurations

Configurations, or patterns, refer to changes in murmur intensity.

Crescendo

A crescendo murmur becomes progressively louder.

Decrescendo

A decrescendo murmur becomes progressively softer.

Crescendo-decrescendo

A crescendo-decrescendo murmur (also called diamond-shaped hair) peaks in intensity and then decreases again.

Plateau-shaped

A plateau-shaped murmur remains equal in intensity.

Bruits

A murmurlike sound of vascular (rather than cardiac) origin is called a *bruit*. If you hear a bruit during arterial auscultation, the patient may have occlusive arterial disease or an arteriovenous fistula. A carotid bruit may suggest carotid artery stenosis. Various high cardiac output conditions—such as anemia, hyperthyroidism, and pheochromocytoma—may also cause bruits.

Vascular abnormalities

outside the norm

Vascular ulcers

Venous ulcers

Venous ulcers result from venous hypertension. These ulcers, the most commonly occurring lower leg ulcers, are typically found around the ankle, as shown.

Lymphatic ulcers

Lymphatic ulcers result from lymphedema, in which the capillaries are compressed by thickened tissue, which occludes blood flow to the skin. Lymphatic ulcers are extremely difficult to treat because of the reduced blood flow. This photo shows a patient with lymphedema of the leg and a large lymphatic ulcer.

Note that vascular ulcers differ in appearance and severity, depending on the part of the vascular system that's affected.

Arterial ulcers

Arterial ulcers result from arterial occlusive disease caused by insufficient blood flow to tissue due to arterial insufficiency. They're commonly found at the distal ends of arterial branches, especially at the tips of the toes, the corners of nail beds, or over bony prominences, as shown.

Able to label?

Identify the arteries that can be palpated for peripheral pulses.

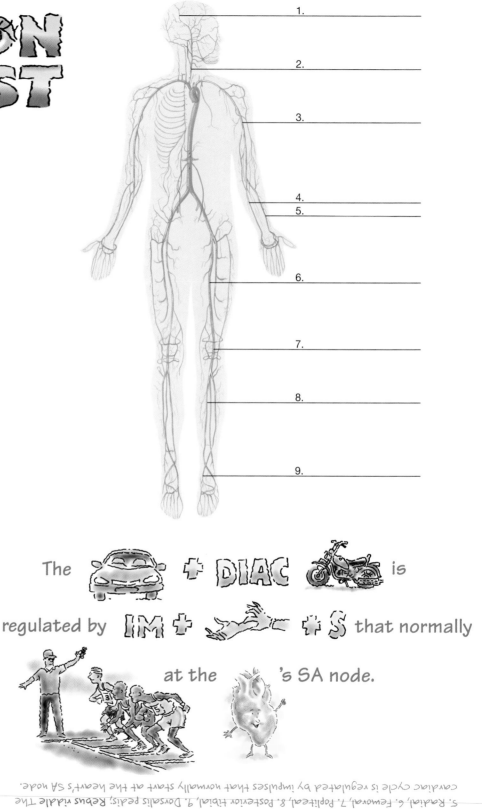

1. _____
2. _____
3. _____
4. _____
5. _____
6. _____
7. _____
8. _____
9. _____

Rebus riddle

Sound out each group of pictures and symbols to reveal information about normal physiology of the heart.

The [car] + DIAC [motorcycle] is regulated by IM + [hand] + S that normally [runners] at the [heart]'s SA node.

7

Breasts and axillae

Assessing the axillae can be the pits. Get it? "The pits"?

Anatomy

The breasts, also called *mammary glands* in women, lie on the anterior chest wall. They're located vertically between the second or third and the sixth or seventh ribs over the pectoralis major muscle and the serratus anterior muscle, and horizontally between the sternal border and the midaxillary line.

Breast structures

Each breast has a centrally located nipple of pigmented erectile tissue ringed by an areola that's darker than the adjacent tissue. Sebaceous glands, also called *Montgomery's tubercles*, are scattered on the areola surface, along with hair follicles.

Although we tend to focus on assessing the female breast, don't ignore this part of an assessment in male patients. In men, breast structures include a nipple, an areola, and flat tissue bordering the chest wall.

Differences in areola pigmentation

The pigment of the nipple and areola varies among different races, getting darker as skin tone darkens. Whites have light-colored nipples and areolae, usually pink or light beige. People with darker complexions, such as Blacks and Asians, have medium brown to almost black nipples and areolae.

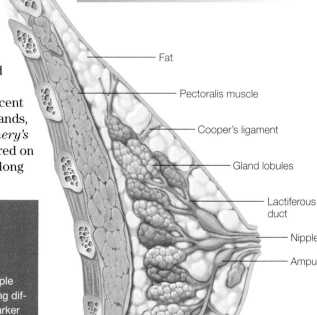

Normal breast anatomy

- Fat
- Pectoralis muscle
- Cooper's ligament
- Gland lobules
- Lactiferous duct
- Nipple
- Ampulla

What lies beneath

Beneath the skin are glandular, fibrous, and fatty tissues that vary in proportion with age, weight, gender, and other factors, such as pregnancy. A small triangle of tissue, called the *tail of Spence*, projects into the axilla. Attached to the chest wall musculature are fibrous bands, called *Cooper's ligaments*, that support each breast.

Support structures of the breast

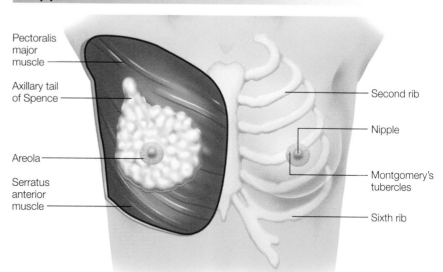

- Pectoralis major muscle
- Axillary tail of Spence
- Areola
- Serratus anterior muscle
- Second rib
- Nipple
- Montgomery's tubercles
- Sixth rib

Lobes and ducts

In women, 12 to 25 glandular lobes containing alveoli that produce milk surround each breast. The lactiferous ducts from each lobe transport milk to the nipple.

- Second rib
- Pectoralis major muscle
- Fatty tissue
- Glandular tissue
- Cooper's ligament (fibrous tissue)
- Lobe
- Lactiferous duct
- Lactiferous sinus
- Lobule

Lymph nodes

The breasts hold several lymph node chains, each serving different areas. The pectoral lymph nodes drain lymph fluid from most of the breast and anterior chest. The brachial nodes drain most of the arm. The subscapular nodes drain the posterior chest wall and part of the arm. The midaxillary nodes located near the ribs and the serratus anterior muscle high in the axilla are the central drain-ing nodes for the pectoral, brachial, and subscapular nodes. In women, the internal mammary nodes drain the mammary lobes. The superficial lymphatic vessels drain the skin.

Lymph nodes of the breast and axillary region

In men and women, the lymphatic system is the most common route for the spread of breast cancer cells.

Triceps brachii muscle

Lateral axillary nodes

Central (mid) axillary nodes

Subscapular (posterior) nodes

Teres major muscle
Pectoral lymph nodes

Latissimus dorsi muscle

Serratus anterior muscle

Apical nodes

Infraclavicular nodes

Pectoralis major muscle

Internal mammary nodes

Subareolar plexus

As time goes on

In females, the breasts start to change at puberty and continue changing during the reproductive years, pregnancy, and menopause.

Changes during puberty

Breast development is an early sign of puberty in girls and usually starts with the breast and nipple protruding as a single mound of flesh between ages 8 and 13. Development of breast tissue in girls younger than age 8 is abnormal.

Changes during the reproductive years

During the reproductive years, a woman's breasts may become full or tender in response to hormonal fluctuations during the menstrual cycle. During pregnancy, breast changes occur in response to hormones from the corpus luteum and the placenta.

Changes after menopause

After menopause, estrogen levels decrease, causing glandular tissue to atrophy and be replaced with fatty deposits.

Breast changes through the life span

Before age 8

Between ages 8 and 13

■ The breast and nipple protrude as a single mound of flesh.

During adulthood (having never given birth)

■ Breasts may become full or tender in response to hormonal fluctuations during the menstrual cycle.

During pregnancy

■ The areola becomes deeply pigmented and increases in diameter.
■ The nipple becomes darker, more prominent, and erect.
■ The breasts enlarge because of the proliferation and hypertrophy of the alveolar cells and lactiferous ducts.
■ As veins engorge, a venous pattern may become visible.
■ Striae may appear as a result of stretching, and Montgomery's tubercles may become prominent.

After pregnancy

■ During breast-feeding, a woman's breasts become full and tense and may feel firm and warm.
■ After breast-feeding ceases, breast size decreases, but usually doesn't return to the prepregnancy state.

After menopause

■ The breasts become flabbier and smaller.
■ As the ligaments relax, the breasts hang loosely from the chest.
■ The nipples flatten, losing some of their erectile quality.
■ The ducts around the nipples may feel like firm strings.

Assessment

Inspect the skin of the breast. Check for edema. Note breast size and symmetry. Then, inspect the nipples.

Examining the breasts

Inspection

Inspect the skin of the breast. It should be smooth, undimpled, and the same color as the rest of the skin. Check for edema, which can accompany lymphatic obstruction and may signal cancer. Note breast size and symmetry. Asymmetry may occur normally in some adult women, with the left breast usually larger than the right.

Inspect the nipples, noting their size and shape. If a nipple is inverted, dimpled, or creased, ask the patient when she first noticed the abnormality.

Next, inspect the patient's breasts while she holds her arms over her head, and then again while she has her hands on her hips. These positions may help you detect skin or nipple dimpling that wasn't obvious before. If the patient has large or pendulous breasts, have her stand with her hands on the back of a chair and lean forward. This position helps reveal subtle breast or nipple asymmetry.

Palpation

Ask the patient to lie in a supine position, and place a small pillow under her shoulder on the side you're examining. Have the patient put her hand behind her head on the side you're examining. This spreads the breast evenly across the chest and makes finding nodules easier. If her breasts are small, she can leave her arm at her side.

best picture

Performing breast palpation

Use your three middle fingers to palpate the patient's breasts systematically. Rotate your fingers gently against the chest wall. Make sure you include the tail of Spence in your examination.

Examining the areola and nipple

After palpating the breasts, palpate the areola and nipple. Gently squeeze the nipple between your thumb and index finger to check for discharge.

Breast palpation methods

Three methods may be used to palpate the breasts during a clinical examination: circular, wedged, or vertical strip. According to the American Cancer Society, the vertical strip method is the most effective method to ensure that the entire breast is palpated. Whatever method you use, be consistent and palpate the entire breast, including the periphery, tail of Spence, and the areola.

Circular	Wedged	Vertical strip

Stress with your patients the importance of having regular clinical breast examinations, and make sure they know how to perform breast self-examination.

Identifying locations of breast lesions

Mentally divide the breast into four quadrants and a fifth segment, the tail of Spence. Describe your findings according to the appropriate quadrant or segment. You can also think of the breast as a clock, with the nipple in the center. Then specify locations according to the time (2 o'clock, for example). Either way, specify the location of a lesion or other findings by the distance in centimeters from the nipple.

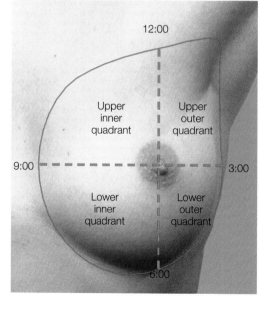

12:00

Upper inner quadrant

Upper outer quadrant

9:00

3:00

Lower inner quadrant

Lower outer quadrant

6:00

Documenting a breast lump

If you palpate a lump, record these characteristics:
- size in centimeters
- shape — round, discoid, regular, or irregular
- consistency — soft, firm, or hard
- mobility
- degree of tenderness
- location, using the quadrant or clock method.

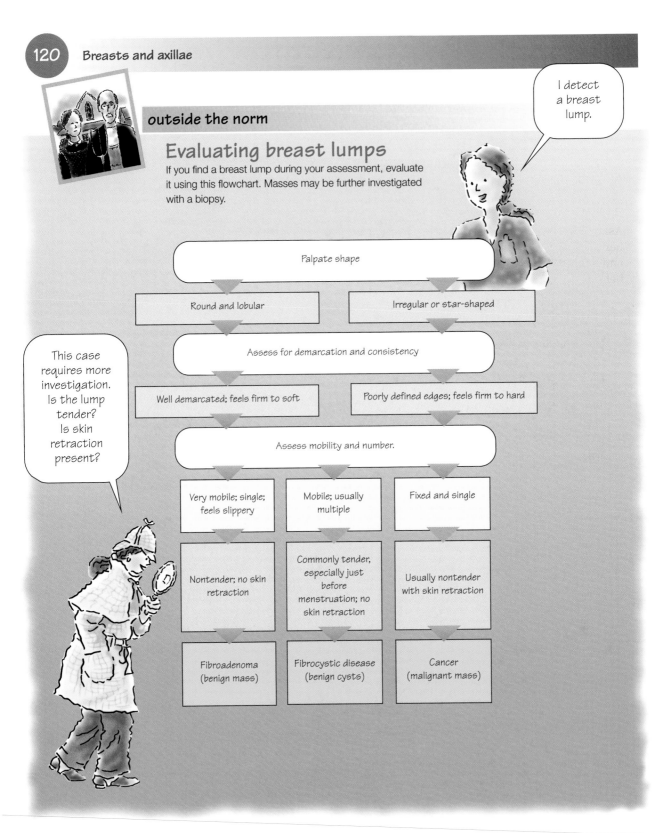

outside the norm

Evaluating breast lumps

If you find a breast lump during your assessment, evaluate it using this flowchart. Masses may be further investigated with a biopsy.

I detect a breast lump.

Palpate shape

Round and lobular | Irregular or star-shaped

Assess for demarcation and consistency

Well demarcated; feels firm to soft | Poorly defined edges; feels firm to hard

This case requires more investigation. Is the lump tender? Is skin retraction present?

Assess mobility and number.

Very mobile; single; feels slippery | Mobile; usually multiple | Fixed and single

Nontender; no skin retraction | Commonly tender, especially just before menstruation; no skin retraction | Usually nontender with skin retraction

Fibroadenoma (benign mass) | Fibrocystic disease (benign cysts) | Cancer (malignant mass)

Examining the axillae

Inspection

With the patient sitting or standing, inspect the skin of the axillae for rashes, infections, or unusual pigmentation.

Palpation

Ask the patient to relax her arm on the side you're examining. Support her elbow with one of your hands. Cup the fingers of your other hand, and reach high into the apex of the axilla. Place your fingers directly behind the pectoral muscles, pointing toward the midclavicle.

Assessing the axillary nodes

Palpate the central nodes by pressing your fingers downward and in toward the chest wall. You can usually palpate one or more of the nodes, which should be soft, small, and nontender. If you feel a hard, large, or tender lesion, try to palpate the other groups of lymph nodes for comparison.

Assessing the clavicular nodes

If the axillary nodes appear abnormal, assess the nodes in the clavicular area. To do this, have the patient relax her neck muscles by flexing her head slightly forward. Stand in front of her and hook your fingers over the clavicle beside the sternocleidomastoid muscle. Rotate your fingers deeply into this area to feel the supraclavicular nodes.

To minimize patient discomfort, warm your hands before palpation.

best picture

Palpating the axilla

- Palpate the central nodes by pressing your fingers downward and in toward the chest wall, as shown.
- Palpate the pectoral and anterior nodes by grasping the anterior axillary fold between your thumb and fingers and palpating inside the borders of the pectoral muscles.
- Palpate the lateral nodes by pressing your fingers along the upper inner arm. Try to compress these nodes against the humerus.
- To palpate the subscapular or posterior nodes, stand behind the patient and press your fingers to feel the inside of the muscle of the posterior axillary fold.

Abnormal findings

outside the norm

Breast cancer mass

Breast cancer findings on palpation include an irregularly shaped mass with poorly defined edges. The mass is fixed, feels firm to hard, and is usually non-tender. Evidence of skin retraction may be present.

Irregular shape with poorly defined edges

> A breast lump, or mass, may be found in any part of the breast, including the axilla.

Ductal carcinoma in situ

Ductal carcinoma in situ is breast cancer in the earliest stage developing in the ducts.

Infiltrating (invasive) ductal carcinoma

Cancer begins within the duct and spreads to the breast's parenchymal tissue.

Dimpling

Breast dimpling—the puckering or retraction of skin on the breast—results from abnormal attachment of the skin to underlying tissue. It suggests an inflammatory or malignant mass beneath the skin surface and usually represents a late sign of breast cancer.

Fibrocystic changes

Fibrocystic changes (benign cysts) are round, elastic, mobile masses that are commonly tender on palpation, especially around menstruation. Multiple cysts may be present. Typically, there's no evidence of skin retraction.

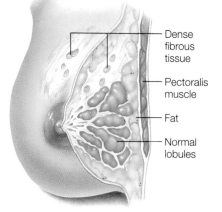

Dense fibrous tissue

Pectoralis muscle

Fat

Normal lobules

Peau d'orange

Usually a late sign of breast cancer, peau d'orange (orange peel skin) is the edematous thickening and pitting of breast skin. This sign can also occur with breast or axillary lymph node infection or Graves' disease. Its striking orange peel appearance stems from lymphatic edema around deepened hair follicles.

Fibroadenoma

A fibroadenoma is a benign, round, lobular, and well-demarcated mobile mass that feels slippery and firm to soft on palpation. It's usually nontender and causes no visible skin retraction.

Rubbery, circumscribed, freely movable benign tumor

outside the norm

Nipple retraction

Nipple retraction, the inward displacement of the nipple below the level of surrounding breast tissue, may indicate an inflammatory breast lesion or cancer. It results from scar tissue formation within a lesion or large mammary duct. As the scar tissue shortens, it pulls adjacent tissue inward, causing nipple deviation, flattening, and finally retraction.

Paget's disease

Paget's disease is a rare form of breast cancer that usually starts as a red, granular or crusted, scaly lesion on the nipple or areola. The lesion may ulcerate and cause erosion of the nipple.

Mastitis and breast engorgement

Mastitis and breast engorgement are disorders that affect lactating females. Mastitis develops when a pathogen in the breast-feeding infant's nose or pharynx invades breast tissue through a fissured or cracked nipple and disrupts normal lactation. The breast becomes tender, hard, swollen, and warm.

Mastitis

Engorgement

Breast engorgement results from venous and lymphatic stasis and alveolar milk accumulation and causes painful breasts that feel heavy and may feel warm.

Keep an eye out for these breast changes, too!

Other breast abnormalities

Nipple discharge

Nipple discharge can occur spontaneously or can be elicited by nipple stimulation. It's characterized as intermittent or constant, unilateral or bilateral, and by color, consistency, and composition. It can be a normal finding; however, nipple discharge can also signal serious underlying disease, particularly when accompanied by other breast changes. Significant causes include endocrine disorders, cancer, certain drugs, and blocked lactiferous ducts.

Breast pain

Breast pain commonly results from benign breast disease, such as mastitis or fibrocystic changes. It may occur during rest or movement and may be aggravated by manipulation or palpation. Breast tenderness refers to pain elicited by physical contact.

Visible veins

Prominent veins in the breast may indicate cancer in some patients; however, they're considered normal in pregnant women because of engorgement.

Male breast concerns

Keep in mind that men also need clinical breast examinations and that the incidence of breast cancer in males is rising. Men with breast disorders may feel uneasy or embarrassed about being examined because they see their condition as being unmanly. Remember that a man needs a gentle, professional hand as much as a woman does.

Male breast cancer

Examine a man's breasts thoroughly during a complete physical assessment. Assess for the same changes you would in a woman. Breast cancer in men usually occurs in the areolar area.

Gynecomastia

Gynecomastia (abnormal enlargement of the male breast) may be barely palpable and is usually bilateral. It can be caused by cirrhosis, leukemia, thyrotoxicosis, hormones, illicit drug use, or alcohol consumption.

Understanding gynecomastia causes

Age-group	Description
Adolescent boys	▪ Temporary stimulation of breast tissue is caused by estrogen. ▪ Adequate testosterone production usually ceases enlargement.
Elderly men	▪ Age-related hormonal alterations and certain medications can cause enlargement.

Able to label?

Identify the breast structures indicated on this illustration.

1. _____
2. _____
3. _____
4. _____
5. _____
6. _____
7. _____
8. _____

Matchmaker

Match the breast palpation technique shown with its correct name.

1. _____

2. _____

3. _____

A. Wedged

B. Vertical strip

C. Circular

8 Gastrointestinal system

This business is great if you can "stomach" the long hours.

Anatomy

The GI tract is a hollow tube that begins at the mouth and ends at the anus. About 25′ (7.5 m) long, the GI tract consists of smooth muscle alternating with blood vessels and nerve tissue. Specialized circular and longitudinal fibers contract, causing peristalsis, which aids in propelling food through the GI tract.

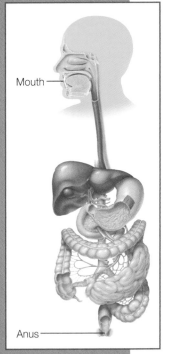

Mouth

Anus

Parotid gland

Mouth

Tongue

Sublingual gland

Submandibular gland

Epiglottis

Pharynx

Trachea

Saliva is produced by three pairs of glands: the parotid, submandibular, and sublingual.

Mouth

■ Begins digestion through chewing, salivating, and swallowing

Tongue

■ Provides sense of taste

Parotid, sublingual, and submandibular glands

■ Produce saliva

Epiglottis

■ Keeps food and fluid from being aspirated into the airway (trachea) by closing over the larynx when food is swallowed

Pharynx

■ Consists of the nasopharynx, oropharynx, and laryngopharynx
■ Allows the passage of food from the mouth to the esophagus
■ Assists in swallowing
■ Secretes mucus, which aids digestion

Esophagus
Descending thoracic aorta
Liver
Stomach
Gallbladder
Rugae
Duodenum
Pancreas
Superior mesenteric vein and artery
Transverse colon
Ascending colon
Descending colon
Small intestine
Ileocecal valve
Cecum
Vermiform appendix
Sigmoid colon
Rectum
External anal sphincter muscles
Anus

Esophagus

- Hollow, muscular tube that's approximately 10" (25.5 cm) long
- Moves food from the pharynx to the stomach using peristalsis

Stomach

- Dilated, saclike structure that lies obliquely in the left upper quadrant
- Contains two important sphincters: the cardiac sphincter, which protects the entrance to the stomach, and the pyloric sphincter, which guards the exit
- Stores food and mixes it with gastric juices
- Passes chyme into the small intestine for further digestion and absorption

Rugae

- Accordion-like folds in the stomach lining
- Allow stomach to expand

Small intestine

- Consists of the duodenum, jejunum, and ileum
- Location of carbohydrate, fat, and protein breakdown
- Absorbs the end products of digestion

Vermiform appendix

- Fingerlike projection that's attached to the cecum

Large intestine

- Consists of the cecum; ascending, transverse, descending, and sigmoid colons; rectum; and anus
- Absorbs excess water and electrolytes
- Stores food residue
- Eliminates waste products in the form of feces

Esophagogastric junction

Esophagus

Gastroesophageal sphincter
- Normally remains closed to prevent the reflux of gastric contents
- Opens during swallowing, belching, and vomiting

Diaphragm

Stomach

It's music to my ears. My rugae help me expand to accommodate large amounts of food and fluid.

A look at digestion

Digestion is the mechanical, chemical, and enzymatic process by which ingested food is broken down and converted into energy.

Food

| Mouth |
| **Chewing** |
| Saliva |

Swallowing

Bolus

Esophagus

Stomach

Digesting

Acids, enzymes, mucus

Chyme

Nutrients → Small intestine

| Body |
| **Absorbing** |

Residue

Water → Large intestine

| Body |
| **Absorbing** |

Waste

Rectum

Anus

Excreting

It's alimentary, my dear stomach!

Accessory GI organs and vessels

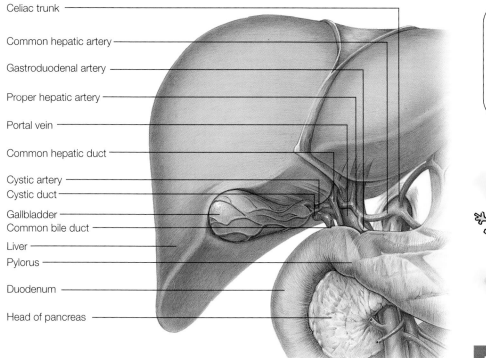

Celiac trunk

Common hepatic artery

Gastroduodenal artery

Proper hepatic artery

Portal vein

Common hepatic duct

Cystic artery
Cystic duct

Gallbladder
Common bile duct

Liver

Pylorus

Duodenum

Head of pancreas

Although I may be the heaviest organ in the body, I only weigh about 3 lb in an adult.

Liver

■ Metabolizes carbohydrates, fats, and proteins
■ Detoxifies blood
■ Converts ammonia to urea for excretion
■ Synthesizes plasma proteins, nonessential amino acids, vitamins, and essential nutrients
■ Secretes bile, a greenish fluid that helps digest fats and absorb fatty acids, cholesterol, and other lipids and gives stools their color

Gallbladder

■ Stores bile from the liver until the bile empties into the duodenum

Bile ducts

■ Hepatic ducts: drain bile from the liver
■ Cystic duct: drains bile from the gallbladder
■ Common bile duct: receives bile from the hepatic and cystic ducts and empties bile into the duodenum

Pancreas

■ Measures 6″ to 8″ (15 to 20.5 cm) in length
■ Consists of a head, body, and tail
■ Releases insulin and glycogen into the bloodstream and produces enzymes that aid in digestion

Vessels

The abdominal aorta supplies blood to the GI tract. It enters the abdomen, separates into the common iliac arteries, and then branches into many arteries that extend the length of the GI tract.

The gastric and splenic veins drain absorbed nutrients into the portal vein of the liver. After entering the liver, the venous blood circulates and then exits the liver through the hepatic vein, emptying into the inferior vena cava.

Assessment

Assessing the abdomen

Use inspection, auscultation, percussion, and palpation to examine the abdomen. Begin by mentally dividing the abdomen into four areas: the right upper quadrant (RUQ), left upper quadrant (LUQ), right lower quadrant (RLQ), and left lower quadrant (LLQ).

Abdominal quadrants and their structures

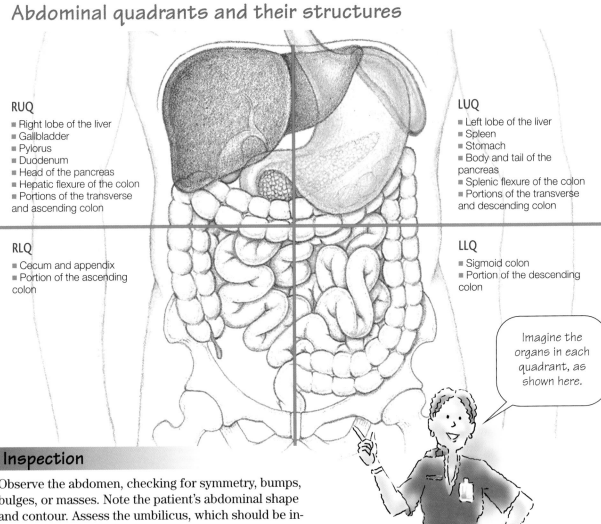

RUQ

- Right lobe of the liver
- Gallbladder
- Pylorus
- Duodenum
- Head of the pancreas
- Hepatic flexure of the colon
- Portions of the transverse and ascending colon

LUQ

- Left lobe of the liver
- Spleen
- Stomach
- Body and tail of the pancreas
- Splenic flexure of the colon
- Portions of the transverse and descending colon

RLQ

- Cecum and appendix
- Portion of the ascending colon

LLQ

- Sigmoid colon
- Portion of the descending colon

Imagine the organs in each quadrant, as shown here.

Inspection

Observe the abdomen, checking for symmetry, bumps, bulges, or masses. Note the patient's abdominal shape and contour. Assess the umbilicus, which should be inverted and located in the abdominal midline.

Auscultation

Lightly place the diaphragm of your stethoscope in the RLQ, slightly below and to the right of the umbilicus. Auscultate in a clockwise fashion in each of the four quadrants. Note the character and quality of bowel sounds in each quadrant.

best picture

Auscultating for vascular sounds

Auscultate the abdomen for vascular sounds with the bell of the stethoscope. Using firm pressure, listen over the aorta, as shown, as well as over the renal, iliac, and femoral arteries.

Vascular sound locations

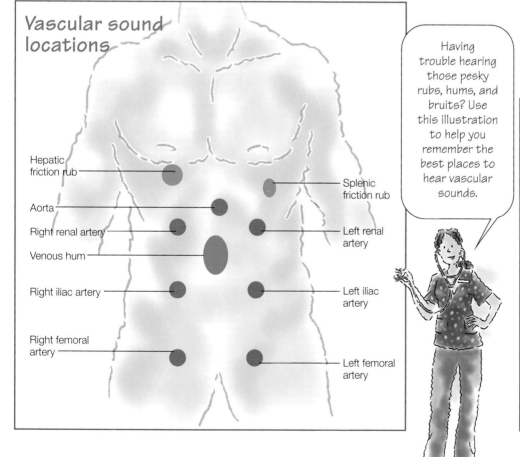

Hepatic friction rub

Aorta

Right renal artery

Venous hum

Right iliac artery

Right femoral artery

Splenic friction rub

Left renal artery

Left iliac artery

Left femoral artery

Having trouble hearing those pesky rubs, hums, and bruits? Use this illustration to help you remember the best places to hear vascular sounds.

What's all the bruit ha ha?

If the patient has hypertension or arterial stenosis, you may hear a bruit—a vascular sound similar to a heart murmur that is caused by turbulent blood flow through a narrowed artery. Occasionally, you may hear a bruit limited to systole in the epigastric region of a healthy person.

Percussion

Direct or indirect percussion is used to detect the size and location of abdominal organs and to detect air or fluid in the abdomen, stomach, or bowel. For direct percussion, strike your hand or finger directly against the patient's abdomen. For indirect percussion, use the middle finger of your dominant hand or a percussion hammer to strike a finger resting on the patient's abdomen. Begin percussion in the RLQ and proceed clockwise, covering all four quadrants. Note where percussed sounds change from tympany to dullness.

> Don't percuss if the patient has an abdominal aortic aneurysm or a transplanted abdominal organ. Doing so can precipitate a rupture or organ rejection.

Drum and humdrum

Normally, two sounds can be heard during percussion of the abdomen: tympany and dullness. Tympany—a clear, hollow sound similar to a drum beating—occurs when you percuss over hollow organs such as an empty stomach or bowel. The degree of tympany depends on the amount of air present and gastric dilation.

When you percuss over solid organs, such as the liver, kidney, or feces-filled intestines, the sound changes to dullness.

Percussing and measuring the liver

Percussion of the liver can help you estimate its size.

best picture

Percussing and measuring the liver

■ Begin percussing the abdomen along the right midclavicular line, starting below the level of the umbilicus.

■ Move upward until the percussion notes change from tympany to dullness, usually at or slightly below the costal margin. This indicates the lower border of the liver.
■ Mark the point of change with a felt-tip pen.
■ Percuss downward along the right midclavicular line, starting above the nipple. Move downward until percussion notes change from normal lung resonance to dullness, usually at the fifth to seventh intercostal space. This indicates the upper border of the liver.
■ Again, mark the point of change with a felt-tip pen.

Estimate the liver's size by measuring the distance between the two marks.

In an adult, a normal liver span is 4 to 8 cm at the midsternal line and 6 to 12 cm at the right midclavicular line.

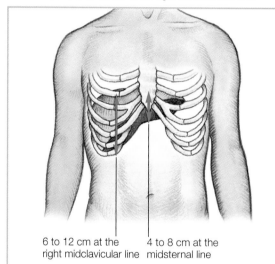

6 to 12 cm at the right midclavicular line   4 to 8 cm at the midsternal line

Percussing the spleen

The spleen is located at about the level of the 10th rib, in the left midaxillary line. Percussion may produce a small area of dullness, generally 7″ (17.8 cm) or less in adults. However, the spleen usually can't be percussed because tympany from the colon masks the dullness of the spleen.

best picture

Percussing the spleen

Percuss the lowest intercostal space in the left anterior axillary line; percussion notes should be tympanic.

Ask the patient to take a deep breath, then percuss this area again. If the spleen is normal in size, the area will remain tympanic. If the tympanic percussion note changes on inspiration to dullness, the spleen is probably enlarged.

To estimate spleen size, outline the spleen's edges by percussing in several directions from areas of tympany to areas of dullness.

Palpation

To perform light palpation

■ Put the fingers of one hand close together.
■ Depress the skin about ½″ (1.5 cm) with your fingertips, and make gentle, rotating movements. Avoid short, quick jabs.

To perform deep palpation

■ Push the abdomen down 2″ to 3″ (5 to 7.5 cm); in an obese patient, put one hand on top of the other and push.
■ Palpate the entire abdomen in a clockwise direction, checking for tenderness, pulsations, organ enlargement, and masses.

The abdomen should be soft and nontender. As you palpate the four quadrants, note organs, masses, areas of fluid accumulation, and areas of tenderness or increased resistance. Determine whether resistance is due to the patient's being cold, tense, or ticklish, or if it's due to involuntary guarding or rigidity from muscle spasms or peritoneal inflammation.

Don't palpate a rigid abdomen. Peritoneal inflammation may be present, in which case palpation could cause pain or rupture an inflamed organ.

best picture

Palpating the liver

Palpate the patient's liver to check for enlargement and tenderness.

Method 1: Standard palpation

- Place the patient in the supine position. Standing at his right side, place your left hand under his back at the approximate location of the liver.
- Place your right hand slightly below the mark at the liver's upper border that you made during percussion. Point the fingers of your right hand toward the patient's head just under the right costal margin.
- As the patient inhales deeply, gently press in and up on the abdomen until the liver brushes under your right hand. The edge should be smooth, firm, and somewhat round. Note any tenderness.

Method 2: Hooking the liver

- Stand next to the patient's right shoulder, facing his feet. Place your hands side by side, and hook your fingertips over the right costal margin, below the lower mark of dullness.
- Ask the patient to take a deep breath as you push your fingertips in and up. If the liver is palpable, you may feel its edge as it slides down in the abdomen as he breathes in.

Practitioners have a choice of two methods for palpating the liver. I wonder which one Sophie would choose.

best picture

Palpating the spleen

Palpate the spleen to detect tenderness and enlargement. Splenic tenderness may result from infections, which are common in a patient with an immunodeficiency disorder.

■ With the patient in a supine position and you at his right side, reach across him to support the posterior lower left rib cage with your left hand.

■ Place your right hand below the left costal margin and press inward.

■ Instruct the patient to take a deep breath. The spleen normally shouldn't descend on deep inspiration below the 9th or 10th intercostal space in the posterior midaxillary line.

■ Normally the spleen isn't palpable. If the spleen is enlarged, you'll feel its rigid border. If you do feel the spleen, stop palpating immediately because an enlarged spleen can easily rupture.

Special assessment techniques

Check for ascites, a large accumulation of fluid in the peritoneal cavity caused by advanced liver disease, heart failure, pancreatitis, or cancer.

best picture

Checking for ascites

■ Have an assistant place the ulnar edge of her hand firmly on the patient's abdomen at its midline.

■ As you stand facing the patient's head, place the palm of your left hand against the patient's right flank, as shown below.

■ Give the left abdomen a firm tap with your right hand. If ascites is present, you may see and feel a "fluid wave" ripple across the abdomen.

■ If you detect ascites, use a tape measure to measure the fullest part of the abdomen. Mark this point on the patient's abdomen with a felt-tip pen so you'll be sure to measure it consistently. This measurement is important, especially if fluid removal or paracentesis is performed.

Then inspect and palpate the abdominal aorta.

Perform the test for rebound tenderness and iliopsoas and obturator sign when you suspect peritoneal inflammation. Perform these assessment techniques at the end of your abdominal examination.

best picture

Assessing the abdominal aorta

■ Inspect the abdomen for aortic pulsations, which may indicate an aortic aneurysm. Don't palpate a suspected aortic aneurysm because of the risk of rupture.

■ If no visible pulsatile mass is visible, palpate the upper abdomen to the left of the midline for the aortic pulsation, as shown. Normally, the aortic pulsation is regular and moderately strong.

■ In patients older than age 50, assess the width of the aorta by pressing firmly into the upper abdomen with one hand on each side of the aorta. The width of the normal aorta should be less than 1¼" (3 cm).

Eliciting rebound tenderness in children

Eliciting rebound tenderness in young children who can't verbalize how they feel may be difficult. Be alert for such clues as an anguished facial expression, a grimace, or intensified crying.

When attempting to assess this symptom, use techniques that elicit minimal tenderness. For example, have the child hop or jump to allow tissue to rebound gently while you watch closely for signs of pain. With this technique, the child won't associate the exacerbation of his pain with your actions, and you may gain the child's cooperation.

Eliciting abdominal pain

Rebound tenderness and the iliopsoas and obturator signs can indicate such conditions as appendicitis and peritonitis.

Rebound tenderness

■ Help the patient into a supine position with his knees flexed to relax the abdominal muscles.
■ Place your hands gently on the right lower quadrant at McBurney's point (located about midway between the umbilicus and the anterior superior iliac spine).
■ Slowly and deeply dip your fingers into the area; then release the pressure in a quick, smooth motion.
■ Pain on release—rebound tenderness—is a positive sign. The pain may radiate to the umbilicus.

Iliopsoas sign

■ Help the patient into a supine position with his legs straight.
■ Instruct him to raise his right leg upward as you exert slight downward pressure with your hand on his right thigh.
■ Repeat the maneuver with the left leg.
■ When testing either leg, increased abdominal pain is a positive result, indicating irritation of the psoas muscle.

Obturator sign

■ Help the patient into a supine position with his right leg flexed 90 degrees at the hip and knee.
■ Hold the leg just above the knee and at the ankle; then rotate the leg laterally and medially.
■ Pain in the hypogastric region is a positive sign, indicating irritation of the obturator muscle.

To minimize the risk of rupturing an inflamed appendix, don't repeat the maneuver for assessing rebound tenderness.

Caution

Examining the rectum and anus

If your patient is age 40 or older, perform a rectal examination as part of your GI assessment. Be sure to explain the procedure to the patient before you begin.

Inspection

Put on gloves and spread the buttocks to expose the anus and surrounding tissue. The skin in the perianal area is normally somewhat darker than that of the surrounding area. Check for fissures, lesions, scars, inflammation, discharge, rectal prolapse, and external hemorrhoids. Then ask the patient to strain as if he's having a bowel movement. This action may reveal internal hemorrhoids, polyps, or fissures.

Palpation

Apply a water-soluble lubricant to your gloved index finger. Tell the patient to relax and warn him that he'll feel some pressure. Ask the patient to bear down. As the sphincter opens, gently insert your finger into the rectum, toward the umbilicus. To palpate as much of the rectal wall as possible, rotate your finger clockwise and then counterclockwise. The rectal walls should feel soft and smooth, without masses, fecal impaction, or tenderness.

Remove your finger from the rectum, and inspect the glove for stool, blood, and mucus. Test fecal matter adhering to the glove for occult blood using a guaiac test.

If your patient has problems with his rectum, use your inspection and palpation skills to detect them.

Abnormal findings

outside the norm

Abdominal distention

Distention may result from gas, a tumor, or a colon filled with feces. It may also be caused by an incisional hernia, which may protrude when the patient lifts his head and shoulders.

Gas

Incisional hernia

Tumor

Abdominal pain

Abdominal pain may indicate ulcers, intestinal obstruction, appendicitis, cholecystitis, peritonitis, or other inflammatory disorders. For example, a duodenal ulcer can cause gnawing abdominal pain in the midepigastrium 1½ to 3 hours after the patient has eaten.

If your patient complains of abdominal pain, ask him to describe the pain and when it started. As shown in the table below, the type of pain is a clue to its possible cause.

Type of abdominal pain	Possible cause
Burning	▪ Peptic ulcer ▪ Gastroesophageal reflux disease
Cramping	▪ Biliary colic ▪ Irritable bowel syndrome ▪ Diarrhea ▪ Constipation ▪ Flatulence
Severe cramping	▪ Appendicitis ▪ Crohn's disease ▪ Diverticulitis
Stabbing	▪ Pancreatitis ▪ Cholecystitis

Abdominal pain origins

After you assess the location of a patient's pain, use this chart to get an idea of the most likely source of the pain.

Affected organ	Visceral pain	Parietal pain	Referred pain
Stomach	Midepigastrium	Midepigastrium and left upper quadrant	Shoulders
Small intestine	Periumbilical area	Over affected site	Midback (rare)
Appendix	Periumbilical area	Right lower quadrant	Right lower quadrant
Proximal colon	Periumbilical area and right flank for ascending colon	Over affected site	Right lower quadrant and back (rare)
Distal colon	Hypogastrium and left flank for descending colon	Over affected site	Left lower quadrant and back (rare)
Gallbladder	Midepigastrium	Right upper quadrant	Right subscapular area
Ureters	Costovertebral angle	Over affected site	Groin; scrotum in men, labia in women (rare)
Pancreas	Midepigastrium and left upper quadrant	Midepigastrium and left upper quadrant	Back and left shoulder
Ovaries, fallopian tubes, and uterus	Hypogastrium and groin	Over affected site	Inner thighs

take note

Documenting abdominal pain

2/19/2006	1345	Pt. admitted to emergency department at 1330 c/o burning LUQ abdominal pain rated as 5 on 0 to 10 scale. Episode of vomiting x 1, approx. 200 ml of coffee-ground emesis. LUQ tenderness on palpation, no distention, no abdominal bruits. Bowels sounds heard in all four quadrants. Skin cool and dry, color pale, lips and nail beds pink. I.V. started in left hand with #16 gauge angiocath and 1,000 ml D₅NSS infusing at 125 ml/hour. Lab work drawn. Dr. Labonte in at 1335, and CT scan of the abdomen scheduled for 1400. ————————————————Antoinette Stewart, RN

outside the norm

Abnormal abdominal sounds

Sound and description	Location	Possible cause
Abnormal bowel sounds		
Hyperactive sounds (unrelated to hunger)	Any quadrant	Diarrhea, laxative use, or early intestinal obstruction
Hypoactive, then absent sounds	Any quadrant	Paralytic ileus or peritonitis
High-pitched tinkling sounds	Any quadrant	Intestinal fluid and air under tension in a dilated bowel
High-pitched rushing sounds coinciding with abdominal cramps	Any quadrant	Intestinal obstruction (life-threatening)
Systolic bruits		
Vascular blowing sounds resembling cardiac murmurs	Over abdominal aorta	Partial arterial obstruction or turbulent blood flow
	Over renal artery	Renal artery stenosis
	Over iliac artery	Iliac artery stenosis
Venous hum		
Continuous, medium-pitched tone created by blood flow in a large engorged vascular organ such as the liver	Epigastric and umbilical regions	Increased collateral circulation between portal and systemic venous systems, such as in cirrhosis
Friction rub		
Harsh, grating sound like two pieces of sandpaper rubbing together	Over liver and spleen	Inflammation of the peritoneal surface of liver, such as from a tumor

Skin color changes

Areas of abdominal redness may indicate inflammation. Dilated, tortuous, visible abdominal veins may indicate inferior vena cava obstruction. Other changes include jaundice, icteric sclera, spider angiomas, Cullen's sign, and Grey Turner's sign.

Jaundice

Yellowing of the skin indicates liver or biliary tract disease.

Spider angiomas

Cutaneous spider angiomas—areas of dilated capillaries or arterioles—may signal liver disease.

Cullen's sign

Cullen's sign, a bluish periumbilical discoloration, signals intra-abdominal hemorrhage. It may be seen in acute hemorrhagic pancreatitis, with massive hemorrhage after trauma.

Usually, Cullen's sign appears gradually. Blood travels from a retroperitoneal organ or structure to the periumbilical area, where it diffuses through subcutaneous tissue. The extent of discoloration depends on the extent of bleeding. This sign may be difficult to detect in a dark-skinned person.

Grey Turner's and Cullen's signs may be seen in patients with acute hemorrhagic pancreatitis.

Grey Turner's sign

Grey Turner's sign (also known as *Turner's sign*) is a bruiselike skin discoloration of the flank area. This sign typically appears 6 to 24 hours after the onset of retroperitoneal hemorrhage associated with acute pancreatitis.

Other common GI abnormalities

Bloody stools

The passage of bloody stools, also known as *hematochezia,* usually indicates GI bleeding. It may also result from colorectal cancer, colitis, Crohn's disease, or an anal fissure or hemorrhoids.

Constipation

Constipation can be caused by immobility, a sedentary lifestyle, and medications. The patient may complain of a dull ache in the abdomen, and a full feeling. A patient with complete intestinal obstruction won't pass flatus or stools and won't have bowel sounds below the obstruction. Constipation occurs more commonly in older patients.

Diarrhea

Diarrhea may be caused by toxins, medications, or a GI condition such as Crohn's disease. Cramping, abdominal tenderness, anorexia, and hyperactive bowel sounds may accompany diarrhea.

Dysphagia

Dysphagia, or difficulty swallowing, may be accompanied by weight loss. It can be caused by an obstruction, achalasia of the lower esophagogastric junction, or a neurologic disease, such as stroke or Parkinson's disease. Dysphagia can lead to aspiration and pneumonia.

Nausea and vomiting

Usually occurring together, nausea and vomiting can be caused by existing illnesses, such as myocardial infarction, gastric and peritoneal irritation, appendicitis, bowel obstruction, cholecystitis, acute pancreatitis, and neurologic disturbances, or by some medications.

Hepatomegaly

Hepatomegaly (enlargement of the liver) is commonly associated with hepatitis and other liver diseases.

Splenomegaly

Splenomegaly is enlargement of the spleen. Conditions that cause splenomegaly include mononucleosis, trauma, and illnesses that destroy red blood cells, such as sickle cell anemia and some cancers.

Color my world

In the illustration shown, color the liver brown, the stomach pink, and the gallbladder green.

Matchmaker

Match each of the assessment techniques listed with the image that shows the best way to perform it.

1. _____

2. _____

3. _____

4. _____

A. Liver percussion

B. Liver palpation

C. Spleen percussion

D. Spleen palpation

9
Musculoskeletal system

No bones about it, musculoskeletal assessment is an important part of this production. Roll 'em!

Anatomy

The three main parts of the musculoskeletal system are the muscles, bones, and joints.

Muscles

Muscles are groups of contractile cells or fibers that affect movement of an organ or another part of the body. Skeletal muscles contract and produce skeletal movement when they receive a stimulus from the central nervous system (CNS). The CNS is responsible for involuntary and voluntary muscle function.

Tendons are tough fibrous portions of muscle that attach the muscles to bone.

Bursae are sacs filled with friction-reducing synovial fluid that are located in areas of high friction such as the knee. Bursae allow adjacent muscles or muscles and tendons to glide smoothly over each other during movement.

> Thanks to the bursae, there's less friction between us.

Major muscles of the body

Anterior view

- Deltoid
- Pectoralis major
- Rectus abdominis
- Biceps brachii
- Brachialis
- External abdominal oblique
- Flexor pollicis longus
- Pronator quadratus
- Abductor pollicis longus
- Flexor retinaculum
- Vastus intermedius
- Vastus lateralis
- Vastus medialis
- Patellar ligament
- Soleus
- Tibialis anterior

Posterior view

Occipitalis

Trapezius

Deltoid

Rhomboid major

Triceps brachii

Brachialis

Latissimus dorsi

Gluteus maximus

Biceps femoris

Vastus lateralis

Sartorius

Gastrocnemius

Skeletal muscles move body parts or the body as a whole. They're used for voluntary and involuntary muscle movements.

Bones

The 206 bones of the skeleton form the body's framework, supporting and protecting organs and tissues. The bones also serve as storage sites for minerals such as calcium, and they contain bone marrow, which produces red blood cells.

The skeletal system

Anterior view

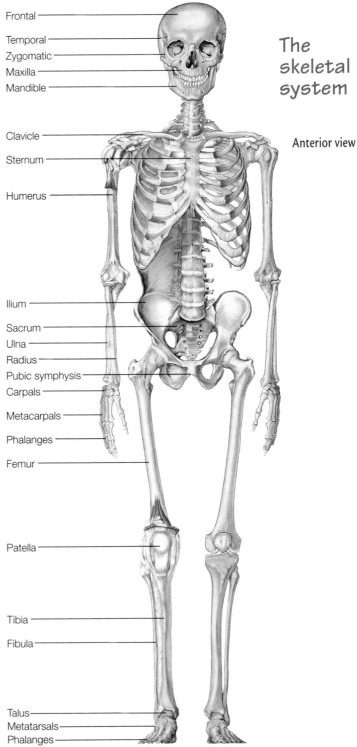

Frontal
Temporal
Zygomatic
Maxilla
Mandible

Clavicle
Sternum

Humerus

Ilium
Sacrum
Ulna
Radius
Pubic symphysis
Carpals
Metacarpals
Phalanges
Femur

Patella

Tibia
Fibula

Talus
Metatarsals
Phalanges

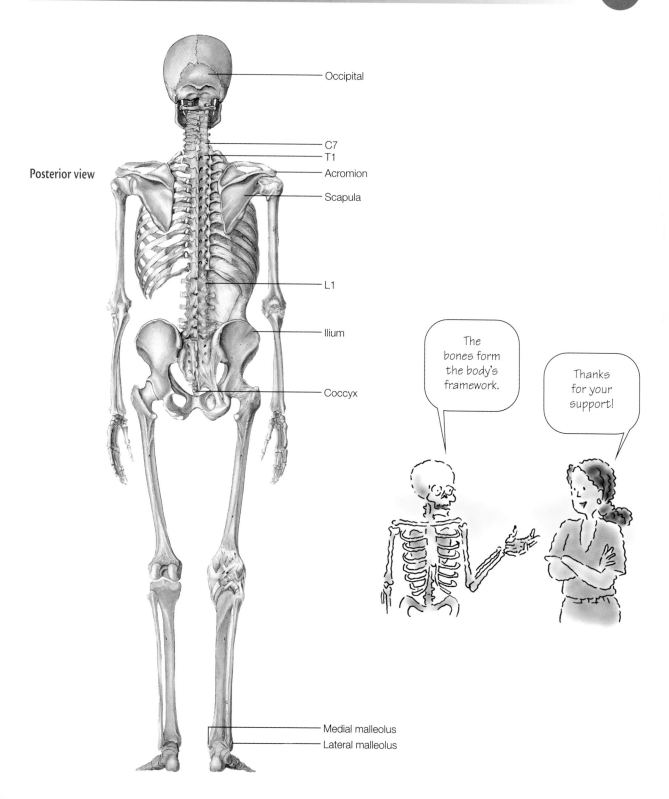

Posterior view

Occipital

C7
T1
Acromion
Scapula

L1

Ilium

Coccyx

Medial malleolus
Lateral malleolus

The bones form the body's framework.

Thanks for your support!

Joints

The junction of two or more bones is called a *joint.* Joints stabilize the bones and allow a specific type of movement. The two types of joints are nonsynovial and synovial.

Nonsynovial

In nonsynovial joints, the bones are connected by fibrous tissue, or cartilage. The bones may be immovable, like the sutures in the skull, or slightly movable, like the vertebrae.

Synovial

Synovial joints move freely; the bones are separate from each other and meet in a cavity filled with synovial fluid, a lubricant. These joints are surrounded by a fibrous capsule that stabilizes the joint structures and surrounds the joint's ligaments—the tough, fibrous bands that join one bone to another.

A look at a synovial joint

Normally, bones fit together. Cartilage—a smooth, fibrous tissue—cushions the end of each bone, and synovial fluid fills the joint space. This fluid lubricates the joint and eases movement, much as the brake fluid functions in a car.

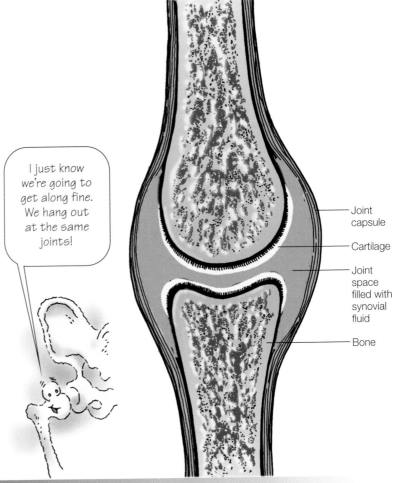

I just know we're going to get along fine. We hang out at the same joints!

Joint capsule

Cartilage

Joint space filled with synovial fluid

Bone

Popular joints

Ball-and-socket joints

- Located in the shoulders and hips
- Allow flexion, extension, adduction, and abduction
- Rotate in their sockets
- Are assessed by their degree of internal and external rotation

Hinge joints

- Include the knee and elbow
- Move in flexion and extension

Types of joint motion

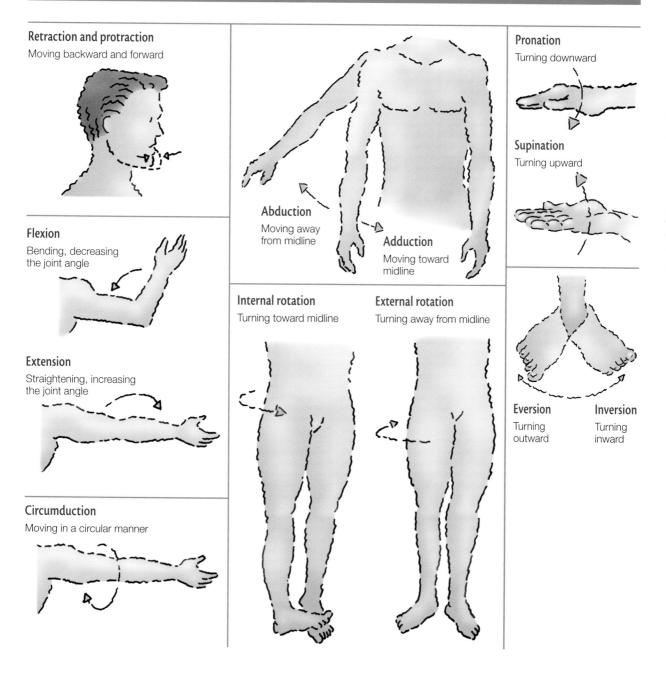

Retraction and protraction
Moving backward and forward

Flexion
Bending, decreasing the joint angle

Extension
Straightening, increasing the joint angle

Circumduction
Moving in a circular manner

Abduction
Moving away from midline

Adduction
Moving toward midline

Internal rotation
Turning toward midline

External rotation
Turning away from midline

Pronation
Turning downward

Supination
Turning upward

Eversion
Turning outward

Inversion
Turning inward

Assessment

You can tell a lot from a patient's walk.

Begin your examination with a general observation of the patient. Note the size and shape of joints, limbs, and body regions. Whenever possible, observe how the patient stands and moves. Watch him walk into the room or, if he's already in, ask him to walk to the door, turn around, and walk back toward you. Then systematically assess the whole body, working from head to toe and from proximal to distal structures.

Assessing the bones and joints

Perform a head-to-toe evaluation of your patient's bones and joints using inspection and palpation. Then perform passive range-of-motion (ROM) exercises to help you determine whether the joints are healthy. Remember, you should never force movement.

Head and jaw

Inspect the patient's face for swelling, symmetry, and evidence of trauma. The mandible should be in the midline, not shifted to the right or left. Then evaluate ROM in the temporo-mandibular joint.

best picture

Evaluating the temporomandibular joint

■ Place the tips of your index fingers in front of the middle of each ear, as shown at right.
■ Ask the patient to open and close his mouth. The patient should be able to open and close his jaw and protract and retract his mandible easily, without pain or tenderness. Your fingertips should drop into the depressed areas over the joints as the patient's mouth opens.
■ If you hear or palpate a click as the patient's mouth opens, suspect an improperly aligned jaw. Swelling of the area, crepitus, or pain may occur.

Neck

Inspect the front, back, and sides of the patient's neck, noting muscle asymmetry or masses. Then palpate the spinous processes of the cervical vertebrae and the areas above each clavicle (supraclavicular fossae) for tenderness, swelling, or nodules. To palpate the neck area:

■ Stand facing the patient with your hands placed lightly on the sides of the neck.

■ Ask him to turn his head from side to side, flex his neck forward, and then extend it backward.

■ Feel for any lumps or tender areas.

■ As the patient moves his neck, listen and palpate for crepitus, an abnormal grating sound. Note that this sound is different from the occasional crack that can be heard from joints.

After inspecting and palpating, check ROM in the neck.

This fella sure has got good range. I don't think he needs to worry about typecasting.

best picture

Assessing neck range of motion

■ Ask the patient to try touching his right ear to his right shoulder and his left ear to his left shoulder. The usual range of motion is 40 degrees on each side.

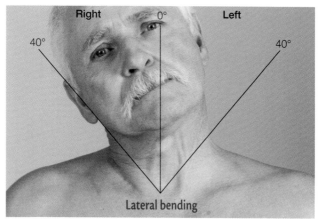

■ Ask him to touch his chin to his chest and then to point his chin toward the ceiling. The neck should flex forward 45 degrees and extend backward 55 degrees.

■ To assess rotation, ask the patient to turn his head to each side without moving his trunk. His chin should be parallel to his shoulders.

■ Finally, ask him to move his head in a circle—normal rotation is 70 degrees.

Spine

Assess spinal position and curvature and the range of spinal movement. Then palpate the spinal processes and the areas lateral to the spine. Have the patient bend at the waist and let his arms hang loosely at his sides. Palpate the spine with your fingertips. Then repeat the palpation using the side of your hand, lightly striking the areas lateral to the spine. Note tenderness, swelling, or spasm.

best picture

Assessing the range of spinal movement

- Ask the patient to straighten up.
- Use a measuring tape to measure the distance from the nape of his neck to his waist.
- Ask the patient to bend forward at the waist.
- Continue to hold the tape at the patient's neck, letting it slip through your fingers slightly to accommodate the increased distance as the spine flexes.
- The length of the spine from neck to waist usually increases by at least 2″ (5 cm) when the patient bends forward. If it doesn't, the patient's mobility may be impaired, and you'll need to assess him further.

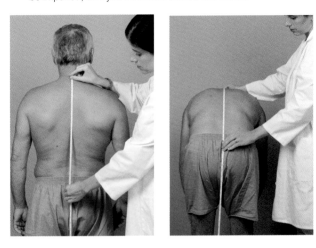

The spine should be in midline position without deviation to either side.

Normal position of spine

Normal curvature of spine

Cervical concavity

Thoracic convexity

Lumbar concavity

When the patient stands in profile, the spine has a reverse "S" shape.

Shoulders and elbows

With the patient sitting or standing, observe the shoulders, noting asymmetry, muscle atrophy, or deformity. Palpate the shoulders with the palmar surfaces of your fingers to locate bony landmarks; note crepitus or tenderness. Using your entire hand, palpate the shoulder muscles for firmness and symmetry. Also palpate the elbow and the ulna for subcutaneous nodules that occur with rheumatoid arthritis. Assess ROM.

Shoulder abduction and adduction

■ To assess abduction, ask the patient to move his arm from the neutral position laterally as far as possible. Normal range of motion (ROM) is 180 degrees.
■ To assess adduction, have the patient move his arm from the neutral position across the front of his body as far as possible. Normal ROM is 50 degrees.

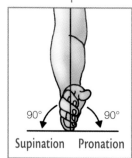

best picture

Assessing shoulder and elbow range of motion

Shoulder flexion and extension

■ To assess flexion, ask the patient to move his arm anteriorly from his side over his head, as if reaching for the sky. Full flexion is 180 degrees.
■ To assess extension, have him move his arm from the neutral position posteriorly as far as possible. Normal extension ranges from 30 to 50 degrees.

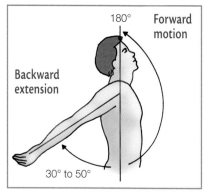

Shoulder external and internal rotation

■ Have the patient abduct his arm with his elbow bent.
■ Ask him to place his hand first behind his head and then behind the small of his back. Normal external and internal rotation is 90 degrees.

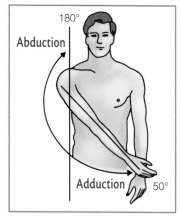

Elbow flexion and extension

■ Have the patient rest his arm at his side.
■ Ask him to flex his elbow and then extend it. Normal ROM is 90 degrees for both flexion and extension.

Elbow pronation and supination

■ Have the patient place the side of his hand on a flat surface with the thumb on top.
■ Ask him to rotate his palm down for pronation and upward for supination.
The normal angle of elbow rotation is 90 degrees in each direction.

Wrists, hands, and fingers

Inspect the wrists and hands for contour, and compare them for symmetry. Also check for nodules, redness, swelling, deformities, and webbing between fingers.

Use your thumb and index finger to palpate both wrists and each finger joint. Note any tenderness, nodules, or bogginess. Then assess ROM of the wrists and fingers.

best picture

Assessing wrist range of motion

Radial and ulnar deviation

■ Ask the patient to rotate each wrist by moving his entire hand—first laterally then medially—as if he's waxing a car.

■ Normal range of motion is 55 degrees laterally (ulnar deviation) and 20 degrees medially (radial deviation).

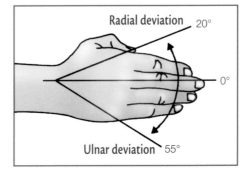

Radial deviation 20°

0°

Ulnar deviation 55°

Extension and flexion

■ Observe the wrist while the patient extends his fingers up toward the ceiling and down toward the floor, as if he's flapping his hand. He should be able to extend his wrist 70 degrees and flex it 90 degrees.

■ If these movements cause pain or numbness, he may have carpal tunnel syndrome. Further assessment is needed.

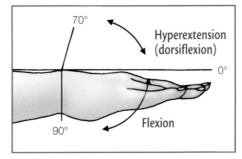

70°

Hyperextension (dorsiflexion)

0°

90°

Flexion

Testing for carpal tunnel syndrome

Tinel's sign

■ Lightly percuss the transverse carpal ligament over the median nerve where the patient's palm and wrist meet.

■ If this action produces numbness and tingling shooting into the palm and finger, the patient has Tinel's sign and may have carpal tunnel syndrome.

Assessing finger range of motion

Extension and flexion

■ Ask the patient to keep his wrist still and move only his fingers—first up toward the ceiling and then down toward the floor.
■ Have the patient make a fist with his thumb remaining straight.
■ Normal hyperextension is 30 degrees; normal flexion, 90 degrees.
■ Ask the patient to touch his thumb to the little finger of the same hand. He should be able to fold or flex his thumb across the palm of his hand so that it touches or points toward the base of his little finger.
■ To assess flexion of all of the fingers, ask the patient to form a fist.

Abduction and adduction

■ To test abduction, have the patient spread his fingers apart.
■ To test adduction, have the patient draw the fingers back together.

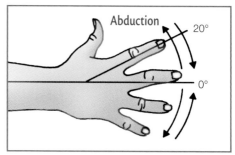

Phalen's maneuver

■ Have the patient put the backs of his hands together and flex his wrists downward at a 90-degree angle.
■ Pain or numbness in his hand or fingers during this maneuver indicates a positive Phalen's sign. The more severe the carpal tunnel syndrome, the more rapidly the symptoms develop.

Hips and knees

Inspect the hip area for contour and symmetry. Inspect the position of the knees, noting whether the patient is bowlegged, with knees that point out, or knock-kneed, with knees that turn in.

Palpate each hip over the iliac crest and trochanteric area for tenderness or instability. Palpate both knees. They should feel smooth, and the tissues should feel solid.

Assess ROM in the hip. These exercises are typically done with the patient in a supine position. If the patient has undergone a total hip replacement, don't perform these maneuvers without the surgeon's permission; motion can dislocate the prothesis. Next, assess ROM in the knee.

best picture

Assessing hip range of motion

Flexion

■ Have the patient lie on his back.
■ Have him bend one knee and pull it toward his abdomen and chest as far as possible.
■ As the patient flexes his knee, the opposite hip and thigh should remain flat.
■ Repeat the test on the opposite side.

Extension

■ Have the patient lie in a prone position (facedown).
■ Gently extend the thigh upward.
■ Repeat the test on the other thigh.

Internal and external rotation

■ Ask the patient to bend his knee and turn his leg inward.
■ Then ask him to turn his leg outward.
■ Normal ROM for internal rotation is 40 degrees; for external rotation, 45 degrees.

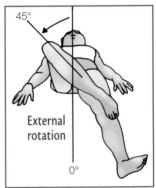

Abduction and adduction

■ Stand alongside the patient and press down on the superior iliac spine of the opposite hip with one hand to stabilize the pelvis.

■ With your other hand, hold the patient's leg by the ankle and gently abduct the hip until you feel the iliac spine move. That movement indicates the limit of hip abduction.

■ While still stabilizing the pelvis, move the ankle medially across the patient's body to assess hip adduction.

■ Repeat on the other side.

■ Normal range of motion (ROM) is about 45 degrees for abduction and 30 degrees for adduction.

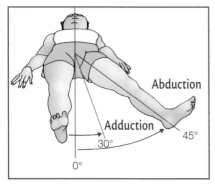

Assessing knee range of motion

■ If the patient is standing, ask him to bend his knee as if trying to touch his heel to his buttocks, as shown. Normal range of motion for flexion is 120 to 130 degrees.

■ If the patient is lying down, have him draw his knee up to his chest. His calf should touch his thigh.

■ Knee extension returns the knee to a neutral position of 0 degrees; however, some knees may normally be hyperextended 15 degrees.

■ If the patient can't extend his leg fully or if his knee pops audibly and painfully, consider the response abnormal. Pronounced crepitus may signal a degenerative disease of the knee. Sudden buckling may indicate a ligament injury.

Assessing for bulge sign

The bulge sign indicates excess fluid in the joint. To assess the patient for this sign, ask him to lie down so that you can palpate his knee. Then give the medial side of his knee two to four firm strokes, as shown, to displace excess fluid.

Lateral check

Next, tap the lateral aspect of the knee while checking for a fluid wave on the medial aspect.

> Checking for symmetry and ROM are key parts of a bone and joint assessment.

Ankles and feet

Inspect the ankles and feet for swelling, redness, nodules, and other deformities. Check the arch of the foot and look for toe deformities. Also note calluses, bunions, corns, in-grown toenails, plantar warts, trophic ulcers, hair loss, or unusual pigmentation.

Use your fingertips to palpate the bony and muscular structures of the ankles and feet. Palpate each toe joint by compressing it with your thumb and fingers. Then assess ROM.

What should I look for in the ankles and feet?

That's easy! Swelling, redness, nodules, or other deformities.

best picture

Assessing ankle and foot range of motion

■ Have the patient sit in a chair or on the side of a bed.
■ Test plantar flexion of the ankle by asking him to point his toes toward the floor.
■ Test dorsiflexion by asking him to point his toes toward the ceiling.
■ Normal range of motion (ROM) for plantar flexion is about 45 degrees; for dorsiflexion, 20 degrees.

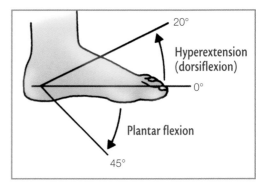

20°

Hyperextension (dorsiflexion)

0°

Plantar flexion

45°

■ Ask the patient to demonstrate inversion by turning his feet inward, and eversion by turning his feet out-ward. Normal ROM for inversion is 30 degrees; for eversion, 20 degrees.

20°   30°

0°   0°

Eversion   Inversion

■ To assess the metatarsophalangeal joints, ask the patient to flex his toes and then straighten them.

Assessing the muscles

Inspect all major muscle groups. Check for symmetry. If a muscle appears atrophied or hypertrophied, measure it by wrapping a tape measure around the largest circumference of the muscle on each side of the body and comparing the two numbers. Note contracture and abnormal movements, such as spasms, tics, tremors, and fasciculation.

Muscle tone

Muscle tone describes muscular resistance to passive stretching. To test the patient's arm muscle tone, move his shoulder through passive ROM exercises. You should feel a slight resistance. Then let his arm drop. It should fall easily to his side.

Test leg muscle tone by putting the patient's hip through passive ROM exercises and then letting the leg fall to the examination table or bed. Like the arm, the leg should fall easily. Abnormal findings include muscle rigidity and flaccidity.

Muscle strength

Observe the patient's gait and movements to form an idea of his general muscle strength. Grade muscle strength on a scale of 0 to 5. Document the results as a fraction, with the score as the numerator and maximum strength as the denominator. Then test specific muscle groups.

take note

Documenting muscle strength

Grading muscle strength

Grade muscle strength on a scale of 0 to 5, as follows:

5/5 **Normal:** Patient moves joint through full range of motion (ROM) and against gravity with full resistance.

4/5 **Good:** Patient completes ROM against gravity with moderate resistance.

3/5 **Fair:** Patient completes ROM against gravity only.

2/5 **Poor:** Patient completes full ROM with gravity eliminated (passive motion).

1/5 **Trace:** Patient's attempt at muscle contraction is palpable but without joint movement.

0/5 **Zero:** No evidence of muscle contraction.

| 3/14/2006 | 1730 | Pt. alert and oriented to person, place, and time. Appetite good — finished 80% of dinner tray. No difficulty swallowing. Feeds self well. Full ROM upper extremities. Strong bilateral handgrip. Weakness in left leg unchanged, muscle strength 3/5 left leg and 5/5 right leg. Son visiting with patient. ———— Mary Petty, RN |

Shoulder, arm, wrist, and hand strength

Test the strength of the patient's shoulder girdle by asking him to extend his arms with the palms up and hold this position for 30 seconds. If he can't lift both arms equally and keep his palms up, or if one arm drifts down, he probably has shoulder girdle weakness on that side.

Next, have the patient hold his arm in front of him with the elbow bent. To test bicep strength, pull down on the flexor surface of his forearm as he resists. To test triceps strength, have him try to straighten his arm as you push upward against the extensor surface of his forearm.

Assess the strength of the patient's flexed wrist by pushing against it. Test the strength of the extended wrist by pushing down on it. Test the strength of finger abduction, thumb opposition, and handgrip the same way.

Leg strength

Ask the patient to lie in a supine position on the examination table or bed and lift both legs at the same time. Note whether he lifts both legs at the same time and to the same distance. To test quadriceps strength, have him lower his legs and raise them again while you press down on his anterior thighs.

Finally, assess ankle strength by having the patient push his foot down against your resistance and then pull his foot up as you try to hold it down.

best picture

Testing muscle strength

To test specific muscle groups, ask the patient to move the muscles while you apply resistance; then compare the contralateral muscle groups. Use the techniques shown here to test the muscle strength of your patient's arm and ankle muscles.

Biceps strength

Triceps strength

Ankle strength: Plantar flexion

Ankle strength: Dorsiflexion

Testing handgrip strength
- Face the patient.
- Extend the first and second fingers of each hand, and ask him to grasp your fingers and squeeze.
- Don't extend fingers with rings on them; a strong handgrip on those fingers can be painful.

Abnormal findings

> Pump up your assessment skills by familiarizing yourself with these abnormal musculoskeletal findings.

outside the norm

Common musculoskeletal abnormalities

Footdrop

Footdrop—plantar flexion of the foot with the toes bent toward the instep—is a characteristic sign of certain peripheral nerve or motor neuron disorders. It results from weakness or paralysis of the dorsiflexor muscles of the foot and ankle. Footdrop may also stem from prolonged immobility.

Muscle spasms

Muscle spasms, or cramps, are strong, painful contractions. They can occur in virtually any muscle but are most common in the calf and foot. Muscle spasms typically result from simple muscle fatigue, exercise, electrolyte imbalances, neuromuscular disorders, and pregnancy.

Muscle atrophy

Muscle atrophy, or muscle wasting, results from denervation or prolonged muscle disuse. Some muscle atrophy also occurs with aging.

Crepitus

Crepitus is an abnormal crunching or grating you can hear and feel when a joint with roughened articular surfaces moves. It occurs in patients with rheumatoid arthritis or osteoarthritis or when broken pieces of bone rub together.

Muscle weakness

Muscle weakness can result from a malfunction in the cerebral hemispheres, brain stem, spinal cord, nerve roots, peripheral nerves, or myoneural junctions and within the muscle itself.

Traumatic injury

Traumatic injuries include fractures, dislocations, amputations, crush injuries, and serious lacerations. To swiftly assess a musculoskeletal injury, remember the 5 P's: pain, paresthesia, paralysis, pallor, and pulse.

Pain

Arm pain (pain anywhere from the hand to the shoulder) and leg pain usually result from musculoskeletal disorders, but they can also stem from neurovascular, cardiovascular, or neurologic disorders.

memory board

The 5 P's of musculoskeletal injury

Pain—Does the patient feel pain? If he does, assess its location, severity, and quality.

Paresthesia—Assess for loss of sensation by touching the injured area with the tip of an open safety pin. Abnormal sensation or loss of sensation indicates neurovascular involvement.

Paralysis—Can the patient move the affected area? If he can't, he might have nerve or tendon damage.

Pallor—Paleness, discoloration, and coolness on the injured side may indicate neurovascular compromise.

Pulse—Check all pulses distal to the injury site. If a pulse is decreased or absent, blood supply to the area is reduced.

outside the norm

Scoliosis

In a patient with scoliosis, lateral deviation of the spine is present and the patient leans to the side. Other findings include:
- uneven shoulder blade height and shoulder blade prominence
- unequal distance between the arms and the body
- asymmetrical waistline
- uneven hip height.

Kyphosis and lordosis

Kyphosis

If the patient has pronounced kyphosis, the thoracic curve is abnormally rounded, as shown below.

Lordosis

If the patient has pronounced lordosis, the lumbar spine is abnormally concave, as shown below. Lordosis (as well as a waddling gait) is normal in pregnant women and young children.

Heberden's and Bouchard's nodes

Heberden's and Bouchard's nodes are typically seen in patients with osteoarthritis, a chronic deterioration of the joint cartilage that commonly occurs in the hips, knees, and joints of the fingers. The nodes may be red, swollen, and painful initially. Eventually, they become painless but are associated with limited joint mobility.

Heberden's nodes

Heberden's nodes are hard, bony, and cartilaginous enlargements that appear on the distal interphalangeal joints.

Bouchard's nodes

Bouchard's nodes are similar but less common and appear on the proximal interphalangeal joints.

Ganglion

A ganglion is a round, enlarged, fluid-filled cyst commonly found on the dorsal side of the wrist. A ganglion may be nontender, but when it develops near a tender sheath, it may be painful and may limit joint mobility.

The more you learn, the more you node.

outside the norm

Rheumatoid arthritis

A chronic, systemic inflammatory immune disorder, rheumatoid arthritis commonly affects bilateral joints of the fingers, wrists, elbows, knees, or ankles as well as surrounding muscles, tendons, ligaments, and blood vessels. Spontaneous remissions and unpredictable exacerbations mark the course of this potentially crippling disease. Swollen, painful, and stiff joints, especially of the hands, are typical in acute rheumatoid arthritis.

As the disease progresses, bone atrophy and misalignment cause visible deformities, restriction of movement, and muscle atrophy. In chronic rheumatoid arthritis, deformities of the interphalangeal joints develop. Swan-neck deformity—hyperextension of the proximal interphalangeal joints with flexion of the distal interphalangeal joints—may occur. A less common deformity is the boutonnière deformity—flexion of the proximal interphalangeal joint with hyperextension of the distal interphalangeal joint.

Gout

Gout is a metabolic disorder in which uric acid deposits in the joints cause the joints to become painful, arthritic, red, and swollen. Skin temperature may be elevated due to the irritation and inflammation.

Boutonnière deformity

Swollen joints

Swan-neck deformity

Acute rheumatoid arthritis   **Chronic rheumatoid arthritis**

Muscular dystrophy

Muscular dystrophy is a group of congenital disorders characterized by progressive symmetrical wasting of skeletal muscles without neural or sensory defects. The most common form is Duchenne's (pseudohypertrophic) muscular dystrophy. Duchenne's occurs during early childhood; onset is insidious and occurs between ages 3 and 5. The disorder initially affects the legs, pelvis, and shoulders. Findings include:

- enlarged, firm calf muscles
- waddling gait, toe-walking, lumbar lordosis, and positive Gower's sign
- difficulty climbing stairs
- history of frequent falls.

Gower's sign

A positive Gower's sign—an inability to lift the trunk without using the hands and arms to brace and push—indicates pelvic muscle weakness, as occurs in muscular dystrophy and spinal muscle atrophy. To check for Gower's sign, place the patient in the supine position and ask him to rise.

Muscles affected by Duchenne's

Deltoid

Pectoralis major

Rectus abdominis

Trapezius

Deltoid

Gluteus maximus

Semitendinous muscles

Biceps femoris

Gastrocnemius

VISION QUEST

Show and tell

Name and describe the assessment techniques shown for testing muscle strength.

1. _____ 2. _____

My word!

Unscramble each of the words. Then use the circled letters from those words to answer the question posed here. *Hint:* The words listed are all related to the muscles affected by this muscular disorder.

Question: What muscular disorder that initially affects the legs, pelvis, and shoulders has an insidious onset that occurs between ages 3 and 5?

1. diedlot _ _ _ _ _ _ _Ⓞ

2. alicesport jarom _ _Ⓞ_ _ _ _ _ _ _ _ _ _ _ _ _

3. azuretips _ _ _ _ _Ⓞ_ _ _

4. useglut summaxi _ _ _ _ _ _ _Ⓞ _ _ _ _ _ _

5. custer biasdimno _ _ _ _ _ _ _ _ _ _ _ _ _ _Ⓞ_ _

6. piesbc semifor _ _ _Ⓞ_ _ _ _ _ _ _ _ _

7. anecgissumrot _ _ _ _ _ _ _ _Ⓞ_ _ _Ⓞ_

8. dothyspry _ _ _ _ _ _ _ _Ⓞ_

Answer: _ _ _ _ _ _ _ _ _ _ , _ _ _ _ _ _ _ _

Answers: Show and tell 1. Biceps strength—The examiner pulls down on the flexor surface of the patient's forearm as the patient resists, 2. Triceps strength—The patient straightens his arm as the examiner pushes upward against the extensor surface of the forearm; My word! 1. Deltoid, 2. Pectoralis major, 3. Trapezius, 4. Gluteus maximus, 5. Rectus abdominis, 6. Biceps femoris, 7. Gastrocnemius, 8. Dystrophy; Question: Duchenne's.

10
Neurologic system

Who are you calling neurotic? Oh wait, that says neurologic!

Anatomy

The neurologic system controls body function and is related to every other body system. It's divided into the central nervous system (CNS), the peripheral nervous system, and the autonomic nervous system.

Cerebrum
- Controls ability to think and reason
- Enclosed by three meninges (dura mater, arachnoid mater, and pia mater)

Thalamus
- Relay station for sensory impulses

Brain stem
- Controls heart rate and rate of breathing

Cerebellum
- Contains major motor and sensory pathways
- Helps maintain equilibrium
- Controls muscle coordination

Hypothalamus
- Controls regulatory functions, including temperature control, pituitary hormone production, and water balance

Lateral view

Dura mater
Arachnoid mater
Pia mater
Skull
Cerebrum
Lateral ventricle
Thalamus
Third ventricle
Brain stem
Cerebellum
Fourth ventricle
Medulla oblongata
Midbrain
Pons
Hypothalamus
Spinal cord
Central canal

You don't have to be a brainiac to remember these three parts. Get it? Brainiac?

Central nervous system

The CNS includes the brain and spinal cord. These two structures collect and interpret voluntary and involuntary motor and sensory stimuli.

Brain

The brain consists of the cerebrum (or *cerebral cortex*), brain stem, and cerebellum. The diencephalon, a division of the cerebrum, contains the thalamus and hypothalamus. The brain stem, which lies below the diencephalon, contains cranial nerves III through XII and regulates automatic body functions, such as heart rate, breathing, and swallowing.

Cerebral lobes and hemispheres

The cerebrum is divided into four lobes and two hemispheres. The right hemisphere controls the left side of the body, and the left hemisphere controls the right side of the body.

Frontal lobe
- Motor control of voluntary muscles
- Personality
- Concentration
- Organization
- Problem-solving

Temporal lobe
- Hearing
- Memory of hearing and vision

Parietal lobe
- Sensory areas for touch, pain, and temperature
- Understanding of speech and language
- Thought expression

Occipital lobe
- Visual recognition
- Focus of the eye

Motor strip

Sensory strip

Frontal lobe

Parietal lobe

Broca's center
- Motor control of speech

Wernicke's center
- Speech interpretation

Occipital lobe

Temporal lobe

Cerebellum

Brain stem
- Midbrain
- Pons
- Medulla

Spinal cord

The spinal cord is the primary pathway for messages traveling between the peripheral areas of the body and the brain. It also mediates the sensory-to-motor transmission path known as the *reflex arc*. Because the reflex arc enters and exits the spinal cord at the same level, reflex pathways don't need to travel up and down the way other stimuli do. The spinal cord extends from the upper border of the first cervical vertebra to the lower border of the first lumbar vertebra. It's encased and protected by a continuation of the meninges and cerebrospinal fluid of the brain. It's also protected by the bony vertebrae of the spine.

Lateral view

Brain

Brain stem

Spinal cord

1
2
3 Cervical
4 nerves
5 (1 to 8)
6
7
8

1
2
3
4
5
6
7 Thoracic
8 nerves
9 (1 to 12)
10
11
12

1
2
3 Lumbar
4 nerves
5 (1 to 5)

1
2 Sacral
3 nerves
4 (1 to 5)
5

Coccygeal nerve

Matter of impulse

The dorsal white matter within the spinal cord contains the ascending tracts that carry impulses up the spinal cord to higher sensory centers. The ventral white matter within the spinal cord contains the descending motor tracts that transmit motor impulses down from the higher motor centers to the spinal cord.

Reflex arc

Spinal nerves, which have sensory and motor portions, control deep tendon and superficial reflexes. A simple reflex arc requires a sensory (or *afferent*) neuron and a motor (or *efferent*) neuron. The knee-jerk, or *patellar*, reflex illustrates the sequence of events in a normal reflex arc:

1. A **sensory receptor** detects the mechanical stimulus produced by the reflex hammer striking the patellar tendon.

2. The sensory neuron carries the impulse along its axon by way of the **spinal nerve** to the **dorsal root,** where it enters the spinal column.

3. In the **anterior horn of the spinal cord,** the sensory neuron joins with a motor neuron, which carries the impulse along its axon by way of a spinal nerve to the muscle.

4. The motor neuron transmits the impulse to the muscle fibers through stimulation of the **motor end plate.** This impulse triggers the muscle to contract and the leg to extend.

Anterior horn of cord

Dorsal root ganglion

Spinal nerve

Sensory nerve

Patellar reflex arc

Motor nerve

Motor end plate

Sensory receptor

Peripheral nervous system

The peripheral nervous system includes the peripheral and cranial nerves:

■ Peripheral sensory nerves transmit stimuli to the posterior horn of the spinal cord from sensory receptors located in the skin, muscles, sensory organs, and viscera. The area of skin that's innervated by each sensory nerve is called a *dermatome*.

■ The 12 pairs of cranial nerves are the primary motor and sensory pathways between the brain, head, and neck.

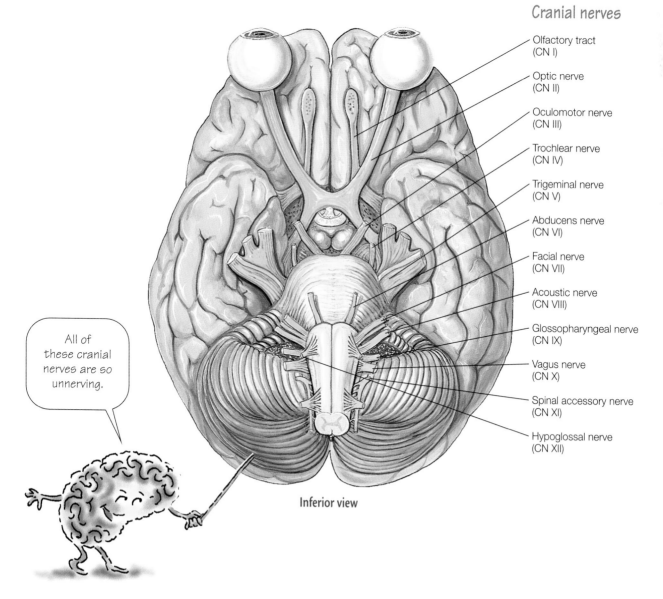

Cranial nerves

Olfactory tract
(CN I)

Optic nerve
(CN II)

Oculomotor nerve
(CN III)

Trochlear nerve
(CN IV)

Trigeminal nerve
(CN V)

Abducens nerve
(CN VI)

Facial nerve
(CN VII)

Acoustic nerve
(CN VIII)

Glossopharyngeal nerve
(CN IX)

Vagus nerve
(CN X)

Spinal accessory nerve
(CN XI)

Hypoglossal nerve
(CN XII)

All of these cranial nerves are so unnerving.

Inferior view

Dermatomes

For the purpose of documenting sensory function, the body is divided into dermatomes. Each dermatome represents an area supplied with sensory nerve fibers from an individual spinal root—cervical (C), thoracic (T), lumbar (L), or sacral (S).

Anterior view

Posterior view

Autonomic nervous system

The autonomic nervous system contains motor neurons that regulate the activities of the visceral organs and affect the smooth and cardiac muscles and glands. It consists of two parts:

■ sympathetic division, which controls fight-or-flight reactions
■ parasympathetic division, which maintains baseline body functions.

Assessment

A complete neurologic examination is long and detailed, and you probably won't perform one in its entirety. However, if your initial screening examination suggests a neurologic problem, you may want to perform a detailed assessment.

Assessing mental status and speech

Mental status assessment begins during the health history. How the patient responds to your questions gives clues to his orientation and memory. Be sure to ask questions that require more than "yes" or "no" answers. Otherwise, confusion or disorientation may not be immediately apparent. If you have doubts about a patient's mental status, perform a screening examination.

Levels of neurologic function

> When assessing the neurologic system, begin with the highest levels of neurologic function and work down to the lowest.

Mental Status & Speech
Cranial Nerve Function
Sensory Function
Motor Function
Reflexes

A quick check of mental status

To quickly screen a patient for disordered thought processes, ask the questions below. An incorrect answer to any question may indicate the need for a complete mental status examination.

> Orientation to time is usually disrupted first; orientation to person, last.

Question	Function screened
What's your name?	Orientation to person
What's your mother's name?	Orientation to other people
What year is it?	Orientation to time
Where are you now?	Orientation to place
How old are you?	Memory
Where were you born?	Remote memory
What did you have for breakfast?	Recent memory
Who's currently the U.S. president?	General knowledge
Can you count backward from 20 to 1?	Attention span and calculation skills

Level of consciousness

To assess level of consciousness (LOC), clearly describe the patient's response to various stimuli.

Alert
- Follows commands
- Responds appropriately to stimuli

Lethargic
- Is drowsy
- Has delayed responses to verbal stimuli

Stuporous
- Requires vigorous stimulation for a response

Comatose
- Doesn't respond appropriately to verbal or painful stimuli

Appearance and behavior

Are the patient's appearance and behavior inappropriate? Is his personal hygiene poor? If so, discuss your findings with the family to determine whether this is a change. Even subtle changes in behavior can signal new onset of a chronic disease or a more acute change that involves the frontal lobe.

Speech

Listen to how well the patient can express himself. Is his speech fluent or fragmented? Note the pace, volume, clarity, and spontaneity of his speech. To assess for dysarthria (difficulty forming words), ask him to repeat the phrase "No ifs, ands, or buts."

Cognitive function

Test orientation, memory, and attention span using the mental status questions on page 177. Note the patient's ability to pay attention.

Content clarity

Assess thought content by evaluating the clarity and cohesiveness of the patient's ideas. Does he use logical transitions between ideas? Does he have hallucinations (sensory perceptions that lack appropriate stimuli) or delusions (beliefs not supported by reality)?

Proverbial test

Test the patient's ability to think abstractly by asking him to interpret a common proverb such as "A stitch in time saves nine." A patient with dementia may interpret this proverb literally. If the patient's primary language isn't English, have a family member ask the patient to explain a saying in his native language, if possible.

Let's say...

Test judgment by asking the patient how he would respond to a hypothetical situation. For example, what would he do if he were in a public building and the fire alarm sounded? Evaluate the appropriateness of his answer.

In the mood

Throughout the interview, note the patient's mood, his emotional lability or stability, and the appropriateness of his emotional responses.

Constructional ability

Observe the patient's ability to perform simple tasks and use various objects. Constructional disorders affect this ability.

Not a numbers person?

When testing attention span and calculation skills, keep in mind that lack of mathematical ability and anxiety can affect the patient's performance. If he has difficulty with numerical computation, ask him to spell the word "world" backward.

Assessing cognitive function includes evaluating the patient's thought content, judgment, and ability to think abstractly.

Assessing cranial nerve function

Cranial nerve assessment reveals valuable information about the condition of the CNS, especially the brain stem. Because of their location, some cranial nerves are more vulnerable to the effects of increasing intracranial pressure (ICP). Therefore, cranial nerve assessment focuses on four 🔑 nerves. Evaluate other nerves if the patient's history or symptoms indicate a potential CNS disorder or when performing a complete nervous system assessment.

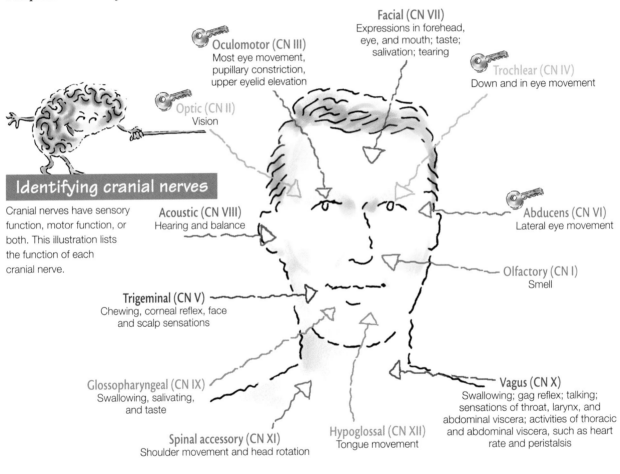

Facial (CN VII)
Expressions in forehead, eye, and mouth; taste; salivation; tearing

Oculomotor (CN III)
Most eye movement, pupillary constriction, upper eyelid elevation

Trochlear (CN IV)
Down and in eye movement

Optic (CN II)
Vision

Identifying cranial nerves

Cranial nerves have sensory function, motor function, or both. This illustration lists the function of each cranial nerve.

Acoustic (CN VIII)
Hearing and balance

Abducens (CN VI)
Lateral eye movement

Olfactory (CN I)
Smell

Trigeminal (CN V)
Chewing, corneal reflex, face and scalp sensations

Glossopharyngeal (CN IX)
Swallowing, salivating, and taste

Spinal accessory (CN XI)
Shoulder movement and head rotation

Hypoglossal (CN XII)
Tongue movement

Vagus (CN X)
Swallowing; gag reflex; talking; sensations of throat, larynx, and abdominal viscera; activities of thoracic and abdominal viscera, such as heart rate and peristalsis

Olfactory nerve

Ask the patient to identify at least two common substances, such as coffee and cinnamon. Make sure the patient's nostrils are patent before performing this test.

Optic nerve

Test visual acuity with a Snellen chart and the Rosenbaum near-vision card. Use confrontation to assess visual fields. Then perform an examination of the optic fundi.

Oculomotor nerve, trochlear nerve, and abducens nerve

Assess these nerves together using the corneal light reflex test, six cardinal positions of gaze, and cover-uncover test (see page 35). Also, inspect the size, shape, and symmetry of the pupils and pupillary reactions to light.

Trigeminal nerve

To assess the sensory component of the trigeminal nerve, ask the patient to close his eyes and then touch him with a wisp of cotton on his forehead, cheek, and jaw on each side. Next, test pain perception by touching the tip of a safety pin to the same three areas. Ask the patient to describe and compare both sensations.

To test the motor component, ask the patient to clench his teeth while you palpate the temporal and masseter muscles. Note the strength of the muscle contraction; it should be equal bilaterally. Then test the corneal reflex.

best picture

Trigeminal nerve assessment sites

Forehead
Cheek
Jaw

best picture

Assessing corneal reflex

To test corneal reflex, touch a wisp of cotton from a cotton ball to the cornea, as shown. The patient should blink. If he doesn't, he may have suffered damage to the sensory fibers of cranial nerve V or to the motor fibers controlled by cranial nerve VII.

Remember, use a wisp of cotton for this test. Even though a 4″ × 4″ gauze pad or tissue is soft, it can cause corneal irritation or abrasions.

Facial nerve

To assess the sensory component, test taste by placing items with various tastes on the anterior portion of the patient's tongue—for example, sugar (sweet), salt, lemon juice (sour), and quinine (bitter). Assess motor function as described at right.

Acoustic nerve

To assess this nerve, use Weber's test and the Rinne test (see pages 40 and 41).

best picture

Testing motor function of the facial nerve

To test motor function, observe the patient's face for symmetry at rest and while he smiles, frowns, and raises his eyebrows. Then have the patient close both eyes tightly. Test muscle strength by attempting to open his eyes, as shown.

Glossopharyngeal nerve and vagus nerve

The glossopharyngeal nerve and the vagus nerve are tested together because their innervation overlaps in the pharynx. Listen to the patient's voice. Then check his gag reflex by touching the tip of a tongue blade against his posterior pharynx and asking him to open wide and say "ah." Watch for the symmetrical upward movement of the soft palate and uvula and for the midline position of the uvula.

Spinal accessory nerve

Assess the spinal accessory nerve by testing the strength of the sternocleidomastoid muscles and the upper portion of the trapezius muscle.

Hypoglossal nerve

Observe the patient's tongue for symmetry. The tongue should be midline, without tremors or fasciculations. Test tongue strength by asking the patient to push his tongue against his cheek as you apply resistance.

best picture

Testing muscle strength

■ Place your palm against the patient's cheek.
■ Ask the patient to turn his head against your resistance, as shown.
■ Place your hands on the patient's shoulder and ask him to shrug his shoulders against your resistance.
■ Repeat each test on the other side, comparing muscle strength.

Assessing sensory function

Pain

Have the patient close his eyes; then touch all the major dermatomes, first with the sharp end of a safety pin and then with the dull end. Proceed in this order: ❶ fingers, ❷ shoulders, ❸ toes, ❹ thighs, and ❺ trunk. Ask him to identify when he feels the sharp stimulus.

If the patient has major deficits, start in the area with the least sensation and move toward the area with the most sensation to help you determine the level of deficit.

Light touch

To test for the sense of light touch, follow the same routine as above but use a wisp of cotton. A patient with a peripheral neuropathy might retain his sensation for light touch after he has lost pain sensation.

Vibration

Apply a vibrating tuning fork over bony prominences while the patient keeps his eyes closed. Start at the distal interphalangeal joint of the index finger and move proximally. Then repeat the test over the interphalangeal joint of the big toe. Test only until the patient feels the vibration because everything above that level will be intact. If vibratory sense is intact, you won't have to check position sense because the same pathway carries both senses.

best picture

Evaluating vibratory sense

To evaluate vibratory sense, apply the base of a vibrating tuning fork to the interphalangeal joint of the patient's great toe, as shown.

Ask him what he feels. If he feels the sensation, he'll typically report a feeling of buzzing or vibration. If he doesn't feel the sensation at the toe, try the medial malleolus. Then continue moving proximally until he feels the sensation. Note where he feels it, and then repeat the process on the other leg.

Position

To be tested for position sense, the patient needs intact vestibular and cerebellar function.

best picture

Assessing position sense

Ask the patient to close his eyes. Then grasp the sides of his big toe, move the toe up and down, and ask him what position it's in. To test the patient's upper extremities, grasp the sides of his index finger and move it back and forth.

Discrimination

Discrimination testing assesses the ability of the cerebral cortex to interpret and integrate information. *Stereognosis* is the ability to discriminate the shape, size, weight, texture, and form of an object by touching and manipulating it.

best picture

Assessing discrimination

Ask the patient to close his eyes and open his hand. Place a common object, such as a key, in his hand and ask him to identify it. If he can't identify the object, test graphesthesia—the ability to recognize figures or numbers written on the skin. Have the patient keep his eyes closed and hold out his hand while you trace a large number on the palm, as shown. Ask him to identify the number.

Assessing motor function

To assess motor function, inspect the muscles and test muscle tone and strength. Also conduct cerebellar testing because the cerebellum plays a role in smooth-muscle movements, such as tics, tremors, and fasciculations.

> Cerebellar testing looks at the patient's coordination and balance.

Muscle tone

To test arm muscle tone, move the patient's shoulder through passive range-of-motion (ROM) exercises. You should feel a slight resistance. Then let the arm drop to the patient's side. It should fall easily.

To test leg muscle tone, guide the hip through passive ROM exercises; then let the leg fall to the bed. The leg shouldn't fall into an externally rotated position.

Muscle strength

Observe the patient's gait and motor activities. Then ask him to move major muscles and muscle groups against resistance.

Cerebellum

If the patient can sit and stand without support, observe him as he walks across the room, turns, and walks back. Note imbalances or abnormalities. A wide-based, unsteady gait indicates cerebellar dysfunction. Deviation to one side may indicate a cerebellar lesion on that side.

Ask the patient to walk heel to toe, and observe his balance. Then perform Romberg's test, as described at right.

1, 2, 3...

To assess rapid alternating movements, ask the patient to touch the thumb of his right hand to his right index finger and then to each of his remaining fingers. Next, ask him to sit with his palms on his thighs. Tell him to turn his palms up and down, gradually increasing his speed. These movements should be accurate and smooth.

Romberg's test

■ Observe the patient's balance as he stands with his eyes open, feet together, and arms at his sides.
■ Ask him to close his eyes.
■ Hold your arms out on either side of him to protect him if he sways.
■ If he falls to one side, the result of Romberg's test is positive.

Assessing reflexes

Evaluating reflexes involves testing deep tendon and superficial reflexes and observing for primitive reflexes, such as grasp and sucking reflexes.

Deep tendon reflexes

Test deep tendon reflexes by moving from head to toe and comparing side to side.

best picture

Biceps reflex

Position the patient's arm so his elbow is flexed at a 45-degree angle and his arm is relaxed. Place your thumb or index finger over the biceps tendon. Strike your finger with the pointed end of the reflex hammer, and watch and feel for the contraction of the biceps muscle and flexion of the forearm.

Triceps reflex

Ask the patient to adduct his arm and place his forearm across his chest. Strike the triceps tendon about 2″ (5 cm) above the olecranon process on the extensor surface of the upper arm. Watch for contraction of the triceps muscle and extension of the forearm.

Brachioradialis reflex

Ask the patient to rest the ulnar surface of his hand on his abdomen or lap with the elbow partially flexed. Strike the radius, and watch for supination of the hand and flexion of the forearm at the elbow.

Patellar reflex

Ask the patient to sit with his legs dangling freely. If he can't sit up, flex his knee at a 45-degree angle and place your nondominant hand behind it for support. Strike the patellar tendon just below the patella, and look for contraction of the quadriceps muscle in the thigh with extension of the leg.

Achilles reflex

Ask the patient to flex his foot. Strike the Achilles tendon, and watch for plantar flexion of the foot at the ankle.

Making the grade

Grade deep tendon reflexes using this scale.

0 =	**Absent impulses**
+1 =	**Diminished impulses**
+2 =	**Normal impulses**
+3 =	**Increased impulses**
+4 =	**Hyperactive impulses**

Superficial reflexes

Stimulating the skin or mucous membranes is a method of testing superficial reflexes. Because superficial reflexes are cutaneous reflexes, the more you try to elicit them in succession, the less of a response you'll get. Carefully observe for a response the first time you stimulate. Assess for plantar response and abdominal reflexes.

Test the abdominal reflexes with the patient in the supine position with his arms at his sides and his knees slightly flexed. Briskly stroke both sides of the abdomen above and below the umbilicus, moving from the periphery toward the midline. Movement of the umbilicus toward the stimulus is normal.

In men, also assess for the cremasteric reflex. Use an applicator stick to stimulate the inner thigh. Normal reaction is contraction of the cremaster muscle and elevation of the testicle on the side of the stimulus.

best picture

Testing for plantar response

To test for plantar response, use an applicator stick or tongue blade and slowly stroke the lateral side of the patient's sole from the heel to the great toe. The normal response in an adult is plantar flexion of the toes.

Dorsiflexion or upward movement of the great toe and fanning of the little toes is called *Babinski's reflex,* an abnormal response that may occur with upper motor neuron lesions.

Plantar response

Babinski's reflex

Primitive reflexes

Primitive reflexes are abnormal in an adult but normal in an infant, whose CNS is immature.

Grasp reflex

Apply gentle pressure to the patient's palm with your fingers. If he grasps your fingers between his index finger and thumb, suspect cortical or premotor cortex damage.

Snout reflex

Lightly tap on the patient's upper lip. Pursing of the lip is a positive snout reflex that indicates frontal lobe damage.

Sucking reflex

Observe the patient while you're feeding him or if he has an oral airway or endotracheal tube in place. If you see a sucking motion, this indicates cortical damage. This reflex is commonly seen in patients with advanced dementia.

Glabella response

The glabella response is elicited by repeatedly tapping the bridge of the patient's nose. Persistent blinking indicates diffuse cortical dysfunction.

Primitive reflexes disappear as the neurologic system matures.

Abnormal findings

LOC is the most sensitive indicator of neurologic dysfunction and may be a valuable adjunct to other findings.

Abnormal neurologic findings include altered LOC, cranial nerve impairment, abnormal gaits, and meningeal irritation.

Altered level of consciousness

Consciousness may be impaired by any disorder that affects the cerebral hemisphere of the brain stem. When assessing LOC, make sure that you provide a stimulus that's strong enough to get a true picture of the patient's baseline. The Glasgow Coma Scale offers an objective way to assess the patient's LOC. Decerebrate and decorticate postures are indicators of severe neurologic damage.

Glasgow Coma Scale

A decreased score in one or more of the following categories may signal an impending neurologic crisis. Add the scores for the best response in each category to achieve the total score. A total score of less than 9 indicates severe brain injury.

Test	Score	Patient's response
EYE OPENING		
Spontaneously	4	Opens eyes spontaneously
To speech	3	Opens eyes to verbal command
To pain	2	Opens eyes to painful stimulus
None	1	Doesn't open eyes in response to stimulus
MOTOR RESPONSE		
Obeys	6	Reacts to verbal command
Localizes	5	Identifies localized pain
Withdraws	4	Flexes and withdraws from painful stimulus
Abnormal flexion	3	Assumes a decorticate position
Abnormal extension	2	Assumes a decerebrate position
None	1	No response; lies flaccid
VERBAL RESPONSE		
Oriented	5	Is oriented and converses
Confused	4	Is disoriented and confused
Inappropriate words	3	Replies randomly with incorrect words
Incomprehensible	2	Moans or screams
None	1	No response

outside the norm

Decerebrate posture

In a decerebrate posture, the arms are adducted and extended, with the wrists pronated and the fingers flexed. The legs are stiffly extended, with plantar flexion of the feet. This posture results from damage to upper brain stem.

Decorticate posture

In a decorticate posture, the arms are adducted and flexed, with the wrists and fingers flexed on the chest. The legs are stiffly extended and internally rotated, with plantar flexion of the feet. This posture results from damage to one or both corticospinal tracts.

Cranial nerve impairment

Olfactory impairment

If the patient can't detect odors with both nostrils, he may have a dysfunction in CN I. This dysfunction can result from any condition that affects the olfactory tract, such as a tumor, hemorrhage or, more commonly, a facial bone fracture that crosses the cribriform plate.

Vision impairment

Visual field defects may result from tumors or infarcts of the optic nerve head, optic chiasm, or optic tracts. If the patient's pupillary response to light is affected, he may have damage to the oculomotor nerve. Pupils are also sensitive indicators of neurologic dysfunction.

outside the norm

Visual field defects

Here are some examples of visual field defects. The black areas represent vision loss.

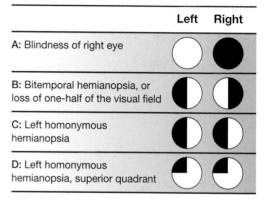

	Left	Right
A: Blindness of right eye		
B: Bitemporal hemianopsia, or loss of one-half of the visual field		
C: Left homonymous hemianopsia		
D: Left homonymous hemianopsia, superior quadrant		

Keeping an eye on pupils

Pupillary changes can unmask conditions that cause damage to or interfere with CN III function.

Small pupils

Small pupils indicate disruption of sympathetic nerve supply to the head caused by spinal cord lesion above T1.

Large pupils

Bilaterally fixed and dilated pupils indicate severe midbrain damage, hypoxia caused by cardiopulmonary arrest, or anticholinergic poisoning.

Midposition fixed pupils

Midposition, or slightly dilated, fixed pupils are characteristic of midbrain involvement caused by edema, hemorrhage, infarctions, or contusions.

One large pupil

Fixation and dilation of only one pupil is a warning sign for herniation of the temporal lobe, which can cause CN III compression. It may also indicate brain stem compression from an aneurysm, increased ICP, or head trauma with subsequent subdural or epidural hematoma.

take note

Documenting pupillary changes

6/5/06	0400	Received pt. from ED with #7 ETT in place, on ventilator with TV 750 cc; Flo₂ 80%; GCS 3; pupils fixed, dilated, and nonreactive to light; BP 100/60 mm Hg; HR 116; RR 22 breaths/min, with no assist. Family at bedside.
		— Brittany James, RN

Other cranial nerve impairments

■ Weakness or paralysis of the eye muscles can result from cranial nerve damage.

■ Damage to the peripheral labyrinth, brain stem, or cerebellum can cause nystagmus. The eyes drift slowly in one direction and then jerk back to the other.

■ Drooping of the eyelid, or *ptosis*, can result from a defect in the oculomotor nerve.

Auditory impairment

Sensorineural hearing loss can result from acoustic nerve lesions. A patient with this type of hearing loss may have trouble hearing high-pitched sounds or may have total loss of hearing in the affected ear.

Speech impairment

Aphasia is a speech disorder caused by injury to the cerebral cortex. Types of aphasia include:

■ *expressive* or *Broca's aphasia* — impaired fluency and difficulty finding words

■ *receptive* or *Wernicke's aphasia* — inability to understand written words or speech and the use of made-up words

■ *global aphasia* — lack of expressive and receptive language.

> Woe is me! All of these abnormal findings are giving me a headache.

Areas of the brain affected by aphasia

Frontal lobe

Broca's center

Temporal lobe

Brain stem

Parietal lobe

Wernicke's center

Occipital lobe

Cerebellum

Abnormal gaits

Gait abnormalities may result from disorders of the cerebellum, posterior columns, corticospinal tract, basal ganglia, and lower motor neurons.

Spastic gait

▧ Stiff, foot-dragging walk caused by unilateral leg muscle hypertonicity

Scissors gait

▧ Adduction of thighs with each step, causing knees to hit or cross in a scissorslike movement

▧ Results from bilateral spastic paresis

Propulsive gait

▧ Stooped, rigid posture

▧ Cardinal sign of advanced Parkinson's disease

Steppage gait

▧ Results from footdrop (usually caused by lower motor neuron disease), which causes outward rotation of hip and exaggerated flexion of knee

▧ Toes hit ground first, producing an audible slap

Waddling gait

▧ Distinctive ducklike walk

▧ Results from deterioration of the pelvic girdle muscles

Meningeal irritation

Positive Brudzinski's and Kernig's signs indicate meningeal irritation, which may occur with meningitis.

Brudzinski's sign

Ask the patient to lie in the supine position. Then place your hand under his neck, and flex it forward, chin to chest. The test is positive if he flexes his ankles, knees, and hips bilaterally. The patient typically complains of pain when the neck is flexed.

Kernig's sign

Ask the patient to lie in the supine position. Flex his hip and knee to form a 90-degree angle. Then attempt to extend this leg. If the patient exhibits pain or resistance to extension and spasm of the hamstring, the test is positive.

VISION QUEST

Able to label?

Identify the cranial nerves indicated on this illustration.

1. _____
2. _____
3. _____
4. _____
5. _____
6. _____
7. _____
8. _____
9. _____
10. _____
11. _____
12. _____

Show and tell

Identify and explain the procedure shown at right.

_____
_____
_____
_____
_____
_____

Answers: Able to label? 1. Optic, 2. Oculomotor, 3. Facial, 4. Trochlear, 5. Abducens, 6. Olfactory, 7. Vagus, 8. Hypoglossal, 9. Spinal accessory, 10. Glossopharyngeal, 11. Trigeminal, 12. Acoustic. Show and tell The procedure shown assesses graphesthesia. With the patient's eyes closed, hold out his hand while you trace a large number on his palm. Ask him to identify the number.

11
Genitourinary system

Your direction will determine how comfortable a patient will be during a GU assessment.

Anatomy

The right kidney extends slightly lower than does the left because it's crowded by the liver. As a result, the right ureter is slightly shorter than the left one.

Renal pelvis
■ Receives urine

Ureters
■ Carry urine from the kidneys to the bladder by peristaltic contractions that occur one to five times per minute

Bladder
■ Hollow and muscular
■ Container for urine collection

External meatus
■ Passageway for urine (and sperm in men)

Aorta
■ Supplies blood to the renal arteries

Urethra
■ Carries urine from the bladder to the outside of the body

Urinary system

The urinary system consists of the kidneys, ureters, bladder, and urethra. The kidneys form urine to remove waste from the body; maintain acid-base, fluid, and electrolyte balance; and assist in blood pressure control.

Each kidney contains roughly one million nephrons. Urine gathers in the collecting tubules and ducts of the nephrons and eventually drains into the ureters, down into the bladder and, when urination occurs, out through the urethra.

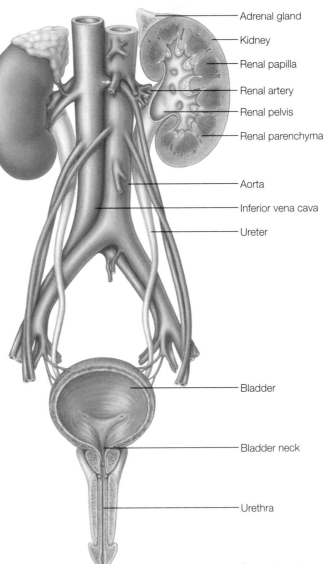

- Adrenal gland
- Kidney
- Renal papilla
- Renal artery
- Renal pelvis
- Renal parenchyma
- Aorta
- Inferior vena cava
- Ureter
- Bladder
- Bladder neck
- Urethra
- External meatus

Female reproductive system

External genitalia

The external genitalia, collectively called the *vulva,* include the mons pubis, labia majora, labia minora, clitoris, vaginal orifice, urethra, and Skene's and Bartholin's glands.

Symphysis pubis
Mons pubis
Prepuce
Clitoris
Urethral orifice
Openings of Skene's glands
Labia majora
Vaginal orifice
Openings of Bartholin's glands
Labia minora
Anus
External anal sphincter

Although most of the female reproductive organs are inside the pelvic cavity, these are external.

Prepuce
- Caps the clitoris

Vestibule
- Contains urethral and vaginal orifices

Mons pubis
- Mound of adipose tissue

Clitoris
- Composed of erectile tissue

Vaginal orifice
- Thin, vertical slit in women who have intact hymens (the thin fold of mucous membrane that partially covers the vaginal opening)
- Large with irregular edges in women whose hymens have been perforated

Labia majora
- Two rounded folds of adipose tissue
- Extend from the mons pubis to the perineum

Labia minora
- Inner vulval lips
- Form the prepuce

Openings of Skene's glands and Bartholin's glands
- Contain ducts that open into the vulva
- Produce lubricating fluids important for the reproductive process

Internal genitalia

The internal genitalia include the vagina, uterus, ovaries, and fallopian tubes.

Uterus

Cervix

Urinary bladder

Urethra

External cervical os

Vagina

Suspensory ligament of ovary

Fallopian tube

Ovary

Cavity of uterus

Abdominal opening of fallopian tube

Cervical canal

Vagina

Uterus

- Hollow, pear-shaped, and muscular
- Divided into the fundus (upper portion) and cervix
- Accommodates the growing fetus during pregnancy

Fallopian tube

- During ovulation, helps guide the ova to the uterus after expulsion from the ovaries

Cervix

- Contains mucus-secreting glands that aid reproduction and protect the uterus from pathogens

Vagina

- Pink, hollow, collapsed tube
- Route of passage for childbirth and menstruation
- Accommodates penis during coitus

Ovary

- Located in the lower abdominal cavity (one on each side of the uterus)
- Produces ova
- Releases estrogen and progesterone
- Fully develops after puberty and shrinks after menopause

Male reproductive system

The male reproductive system includes the penis, scrotum, testes, epididymides, urethra, vas deferens, seminal vesicles, and prostate gland.

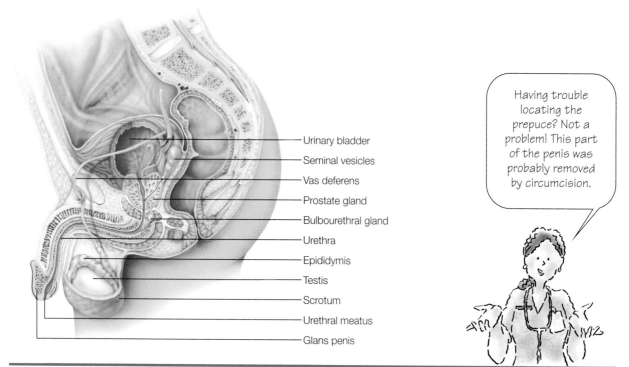

Urinary bladder
Seminal vesicles
Vas deferens
Prostate gland
Bulbourethral gland
Urethra
Epididymis
Testis
Scrotum
Urethral meatus
Glans penis

Having trouble locating the prepuce? Not a problem! This part of the penis was probably removed by circumcision.

Penis

■ Consists of the shaft, glans, urethral meatus, corona, and prepuce (foreskin)
■ Can discharge sperm and semen when erect

Scrotum

■ Loose, wrinkled, deeply pigmented sac
■ Has two compartments, each containing a testicle, an epididymis, and portions of the spermatic cord

Testes

■ Oval and rubbery
■ Produce testosterone and sperm

Epididymides

■ Reservoirs for maturing sperm

Urethra

■ Passage for ejection of sperm and semen during sexual activity

Vas deferens

■ Storage site and pathway for sperm

Seminal vesicles

■ Saclike glands
■ Produce secretions that help form seminal fluid

Prostate gland

■ Produces a thin, milky, alkaline fluid that mixes with seminal fluid during ejaculation to enhance sperm activity

Assessment

Examining the urinary system

First evaluate your patient's vital signs, weight, and mental status. These observations can provide clues about renal dysfunction.

Inspection

Inspect the abdomen with the patient lying supine. The abdomen should be symmetrical and smooth, flat, or concave. Observe the color and shape of the area around the kidneys and bladder. The skin should be free from lesions, bruises, discolorations, and prominent veins.

Percussion

Percuss the kidneys to check for costovertebral angle tenderness that occurs with inflammation.

To percuss the bladder, first ask the patient to empty it. Then have the patient lie in the supine position. Start at the symphysis pubis and percuss upward toward the bladder and over it. You should hear tympany. A dull sound signals retained urine.

Palpation

Because the kidneys lie behind other organs and are protected by muscle, they normally aren't palpable unless they're enlarged. If the kidneys feel enlarged, the patient may have hydronephrosis, cysts, or tumors.

In very thin patients, you may be able to feel the lower end of the right kidney as a smooth round mass that drops on inspiration. In elderly patients, you may be able to palpate both kidneys because of decreased muscle tone and elasticity.

You won't be able to palpate the bladder unless it's distended. With the patient in a supine position, use the fingers of one hand to palpate the lower abdomen in a light dipping motion. A distended bladder will feel firm and relatively smooth, extending above the symphysis pubis.

best picture

Percussing the kidneys

- Have the patient sit up.
- Place the ball of your nondominant hand on the patient's back at the costovertebral angle of the 12th rib.
- Strike the ball of that hand with the ulnar surface of your other hand. Use just enough force to cause a painless but perceptible thud.

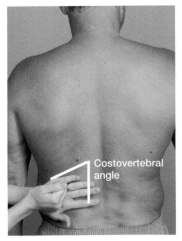

Costovertebral angle

best picture

Palpating the kidneys

Have the patient lie in a supine position. To palpate the right kidney, stand on his right side. Place your left hand under his back and your right hand on his abdomen. Instruct the patient to inhale deeply, so his kidney moves downward. As he inhales, press up with your left hand and down with your right, as shown.

To palpate the left kidney, reach across the patient's abdomen, placing your left hand behind his left flank. Place your right hand over the area of the left kidney. Ask the patient to inhale deeply again. As he does so, pull up with your left hand and press down with your right.

> Remember: Kidneys normally aren't palpable unless they're enlarged.

Examining the female reproductive system

First ask the patient to void. Then have her disrobe and put on an examination gown. Help her into the dorsal lithotomy position, and drape all areas not being examined. Explain the procedure to her before the examination.

Inspecting the external genitalia

Put on gloves. Using your index finger and thumb, gently spread the labia majora and minora. Locate the urethral meatus. It should be a pink, irregular, slitlike opening at the midline, just above the vagina. Note the presence of discharge or ulcerations. Inspect for pubic hair and assess sexual maturity.

The labia should be moist and free from lesions. Normal discharge varies from clear before ovulation to white and opaque after ovulation. It should be odorless and nonirritating to the mucosa.

Examine the vestibule. Check for swelling, redness, lesions, discharge, and unusual odor. Inspect the vaginal opening, noting whether the hymen is intact or perforated.

best picture

Inspecting the genitalia

Palpating the external genitalia

Spread the labia with one hand and palpate with the other. The labia should feel soft and the patient shouldn't feel any pain. Note swelling, hardness, or tenderness. If you detect a mass or lesion, palpate it to determine its size, shape, and consistency. If you find swelling or tenderness, see if you can palpate the Bartholin glands, which normally aren't palpable.

Inspecting the internal genitalia

Nurses don't routinely inspect internal genitalia unless they're in advanced practice. However, you may be asked to assist with this examination.

To start, select an appropriate speculum for your patient. Hold the speculum under warm, running water to lubricate and warm the blades. Don't use other lubricants because many of them can alter Papanicolaou (Pap) test results.

A look at specula

Specula come in various shapes and sizes. Choose an appropriate one for your patient. The illustrations below show a typical speculum and three types of specula available.

best picture

Palpating Bartholin's glands

■ Insert your gloved index finger carefully into the patient's posterior introitus, as shown.
■ Place your thumb along the lateral edge of the swollen or tender labium.
■ Gently squeeze the labium. If discharge from the duct results, culture it.

Parts of a speculum

Anterior blade

Posterior blade

Thumb screws

Handle

Types of specula

Pederson
■ Has narrow blades
■ Used if the patient has an intact hymen, has never given birth through the vaginal canal, or has a contracted introitus from menopause

Graves'
■ Most commonly used

Plastic
■ Disposable
■ For one-time use only

Tell the patient she'll feel internal pressure and possibly some slight, transient discomfort during insertion of the speculum. Encourage the patient to take slow, deep breaths during insertion to relax her abdominal muscles.

best picture

Inserting a speculum

Initial insertion

Put on gloves. Place the index and middle fingers of your nondominant hand about 1″ (2.5 cm) into the vagina. Spread the fingers to exert pressure on the posterior vagina. Hold the speculum in your dominant hand, and insert the blades between your fingers, as shown below.

Deeper insertion

Ask the patient to bear down to open the introitus and relax the perineal muscles. Point the speculum slightly downward, and insert the blades until the base of the speculum touches your fingers, inside the vagina.

Rotate and open

Rotate the speculum in the same plane as the vagina, and withdraw your fingers. Using the thumb of the hand holding the speculum, press the lower lever to open the blades. Open the blades as far as possible and lock them by tightening the thumb screw above the lever. You should now be able to view the cervix clearly.

After inserting the speculum, observe the color, texture, and integrity of the vaginal lining. A thin, white, odorless discharge on the vaginal walls is normal. Examine the cervix for color, position, size, shape, mucosal integrity, and discharge. It should be smooth and round. Then inspect the central cervical opening, or cervical os. Expect to see a clear, watery cervical discharge during ovulation and a slightly bloody discharge just before menstruation.

Obtain a specimen for a Pap test. Finally, unlock and close the blades and withdraw the speculum.

best picture

The normal os

The os is circular in a woman who hasn't given birth vaginally (nulliparous) and a horizontal slit in a woman who has (parous).

Nulliparous

Parous

Palpating the internal genitalia

To palpate the internal genitalia, lubricate the index and middle fingers of your gloved dominant hand. Use the thumb and index finger of your other hand to spread the labia majora. Insert your two lubricated fingers into the vagina, exerting pressure posteriorly to avoid irritating the anterior wall and urethra.

When your fingers are fully inserted, note tenderness or nodularity in the vaginal wall. Ask the patient to bear down so you can assess the support of the vaginal outlet. Bulging of the vaginal wall may indicate a cystocele or a rectocele.

To palpate the cervix, sweep your fingers from side to side across the cervix and around the os. The cervix should be smooth and firm. If you palpate nodules or irregularities, the patient may have cysts, tumors, or other lesions.

Next, place your fingers into the recessed area around the cervix. The cervix should move in all directions. If the patient reports pain during this part of the examination, she may have inflammation of the uterus or adnexa (ovaries, fallopian tubes, and ligaments of the uterus).

If you're in advanced practice, perform a bimanual examination by palpating the uterus and ovaries from the inside and the outside simultaneously.

This procedure is performed by nurses in advanced practice.

best picture

Performing a bimanual examination

During a bimanual examination, palpate the uterus and ovaries from the inside and the outside simultaneously.

Proper position

Put on gloves. Place the index and third fingers of your dominant hand in the patient's vagina and move them up to the cervix. Place the fingers of your other hand on the patient's abdomen between the umbilicus and the symphysis pubis, as shown here.

Elevate the cervix and uterus by pressing upward with the two fingers inside the vagina. At the same time, press down and in with your hand on the abdomen. Try to grasp the uterus between your hands.

Note the position

Move your fingers into the posterior fornix, pressing upward and forward to bring the anterior uterine wall up to your nondominant hand. Use your dominant hand to palpate the lower portion of the uterine wall. Note the position of the uterus.

Rectovaginal palpation, the last step in a genital assessment, is used to examine the posterior part of the uterus and the pelvic cavity. Explain to the patient that this procedure may be uncomfortable. After performing rectovaginal palpation, help the patient to a sitting position and provide privacy for dressing and personal hygiene.

best picture

Performing rectovaginal examination

■ Put on a pair of gloves and apply water-soluble lubricant to the index and middle fingers of your dominant hand.

■ Instruct the patient to bear down with her vaginal and rectal muscles; then insert your index finger a short way into her vagina and your middle finger into her rectum.

■ Use your middle finger to assess rectal muscle and sphincter tone.

■ Insert your middle finger deeper into the rectum, and palpate the rectal wall.

■ Sweep the rectum with your finger, assessing for masses or nodules.

■ Palpate the posterior wall of the uterus through the anterior wall of the rectum, evaluating the uterus for size, shape, tenderness, and masses. The rectovaginal septum (wall between the rectum and vagina) should feel smooth and springy.

■ Place your nondominant hand on the patient's abdomen at the symphysis pubis. With your index finger in the vagina, palpate deeply to feel the posterior edge of the cervix and the lower posterior wall of the uterus, as shown.

■ If stool testing for occult blood is ordered, put on a new glove and apply water-soluble lubricant to your gloved index finger. Slide your index finger into the patient's anus to obtain a small stool sample. Withdraw your finger and test the stool for occult blood using a guiaic test.

■ When you're finished, discard the gloves and wash your hands.

Palpate the walls

Slide your fingers farther into the anterior section of the fornix, the space between the uterus and cervix. You should feel part of the posterior uterine wall with this hand. You should feel part of the anterior uterine wall with the fingertips of your nondominant hand. Note the size, shape, surface characteristics, consistency, and mobility of the uterus as well as tenderness.

Palpate the ovaries

After palpating the anterior and posterior walls of the uterus, move your nondominant hand toward the right lower quadrant of the abdomen. Slip the fingers of your dominant hand into the right fornix and palpate the right ovary. Then palpate the left ovary. Note the size, shape, and contour of each ovary. The ovaries may not be palpable in women who aren't relaxed or who are obese. They shouldn't be palpable in postmenopausal women. Remove your hand from the patient's abdomen and your fingers from her vagina, and discard your gloves.

Male reproductive system

Before examining the male reproductive system, put on gloves. Make the patient as comfortable as possible, and explain all procedures to him.

Penis size depends on the patient's age and overall development.

Inspection

Penis

The penile skin should be slightly wrinkled and pink to light brown in white patients and light brown to dark brown in black patients.

Check the penile shaft and glans for lesions, nodules, inflammations, and swelling. Inspect the glans of an uncircumcised penis by retracting the prepuce. Also check the glans for smegma, a cheesy secretion commonly found beneath the prepuce.

Gently compress the tip of the glans to open the urethral meatus. It should be located in the center of the glans and be pink and smooth. Inspect it for swelling, discharge, lesions, and inflammation. If you note discharge, obtain a culture specimen.

Scrotum and testes

Ask the patient to stand and to hold his penis away from his scrotum so you can observe the scrotum's size and appearance. The left side of the scrotum normally appears lower because the left spermatic cord is longer than the right cord. The skin on the scrotum is commonly darker than the skin on the rest of the body. Spread the surface of the scrotum, and inspect for swelling, nodules, redness, ulcerations, and distended veins.

Inguinal and femoral areas

With the patient still standing, ask him to hold his breath and bear down while you inspect the inguinal and femoral areas for bulges or hernias.

best picture

Examining the urethral meatus

To inspect the urethral meatus, compress the tip of the glans, as shown below.

Urethral meatus

Glans penis

Scrotum

Palpation

Penis

Use your thumb and forefinger to palpate the penile shaft. It should be somewhat firm, and the skin should be smooth and movable. Note swelling, nodules, or indurations.

Testes

The testes should be equal in size, move freely in the scrotal sac, and feel firm, smooth, and rubbery on palpation.

If you note hard, irregular areas or lumps, transilluminate them by darkening the room and pressing the head of a flashlight against the scrotum, behind the lump. The testis and any lumps, masses, warts, or blood-filled areas will appear as opaque shadows. Transilluminate the other testis to compare your findings.

Epididymides

Palpate the epididymides, which are usually located in the posterolateral area of the testes. They should be smooth, discrete, nontender, and free from swelling and induration.

Spermatic cords

Palpate both spermatic cords, one of which is located above each testis. Palpate from the base of the epididymis to the inguinal canal.

If you feel swelling, irregularity, or nodules, transilluminate the problem area. If serous fluid is present, you won't see a glow.

> The palpation step of your assessment is a good time to reinforce the methods for doing a monthly testicular self-examination.

best picture

Palpating the testes

Gently palpate both testes between your thumb and first two fingers of your gloved hand. Assess their size, shape, and response to pressure. A normal response is a deep visceral pain.

Inguinal area

To assess the patient for a direct inguinal hernia, place two fingers over each external inguinal ring and ask the patient to bear down. If he has a hernia, you'll feel a bulge.

To assess the patient for an indirect inguinal hernia, examine him while he's standing and then while he's in a supine position with his knee flexed on the side you're examining.

Femoral area

Although you can't palpate the femoral canal, you can estimate its location to help detect a femoral hernia. Place your right index finger on the right femoral artery with your finger pointing toward the patient's head. Keep your other fingers close together. Your middle finger will rest on the femoral vein, and your ring finger on the femoral canal. Note tenderness or masses. Use your left hand to check the patient's left side.

Prostate gland

Tell the patient that you need to place your finger in his rectum to examine his prostate gland.

best picture

Palpating for an indirect inguinal hernia

Place your gloved finger on the neck of the scrotum and gently insert it into the inguinal canal, as shown below. When you've inserted your finger as far as possible, ask the patient to bear down or cough. A hernia feels like a mass of tissue that withdraws when it meets the finger.

— Inguinal ligament
— Internal ring
— Inguinal canal
— External ring

best picture

Palpating the prostate gland

■ Have the patient stand and lean over the examination table. If he can't do this, have him lie on his left side, with his right knee and hip flexed or with both knees drawn toward his chest.

■ Inspect the skin of the perineal, anal, and posterior scrotal areas. It should be smooth and unbroken, with no protruding masses.

■ Lubricate the gloved index finger of your dominant hand and insert it into the rectum.

■ Tell the patient to relax to ease the passage of the finger through the anal sphincter. If he's having difficulty relaxing the anal sphincter, ask him to bear down as if having a bowel movement while you gently insert your finger.

■ With your finger pad, palpate the prostate gland on the anterior rectal wall just past the anorectal ring. The gland should feel smooth, rubbery, and about the size of a walnut.

Abnormal findings

Urinary system abnormalities

Kidney enlargement

Kidney enlargement may indicate cysts, hydro-nephrosis, or tumors.

Urinary frequency

Urinary frequency is an increased incidence of the urge to urinate. It may be caused by bladder calculi, urinary tract infections (UTIs), and ure-thral stricture. In men, it may be caused by benign prostatic hyperplasia or prostate cancer, which can put pressure on the bladder.

Hematuria

Presence of blood in the urine, or *hematuria*, may indicate UTI, renal calculi, bladder cancer, or trauma to the urinary mucosa. It may also be a temporary condition after urinary tract surgery or urinary catheterization.

Nocturia

Excessive urination at night, or *nocturia*, is a common sign of renal or lower urinary tract disorders. It can result from endocrine or metabolic disorders or prostate cancer. It can also be an adverse effect of diuretics.

Urinary incontinence

Urinary incontinence may be transient or permanent. The amount of urine released may be small or large. Possible causes include stress incontinence, tumor, bladder cancer and calculi, and neurologic conditions, such as Guillain-Barré syndrome, multiple sclerosis, and spinal cord injury.

take note

Documenting kidney palpation

| 5/26/2006 | 0500 | Pt. alert and oriented with c/o right flank pain, nausea, and vomiting. Pt. rates the pain 8/10 on a 0 to 10 pain scale. She reports hematuria, pain on urination, dribbling, and urinary hesitancy. Right kidney is palpable. Vital signs: BP 146/92, HR 110, RR 22, and temp. 100.4° F. Findings reported at 0445 to Dr. Renale, MD. |
| | | ——————————Jane Stephens, RN |

Female genital abnormalities

Syphilitic chancre

In the early stages, syphilitic chancre causes a red, painless, eroding lesion with a raised, indurated border. The lesion usually appears inside the vagina but may also appear on the external genitalia.

Vaginitis and abnormal discharge

Vaginitis usually results from an overgrowth of infectious organisms. It causes redness, itching, dyspareunia (painful intercourse), dysuria, and a malodorous discharge. Vaginitis occurs with bacterial vaginosis, *Candida albicans* infection (a fungal infection), trichomoniasis, and mucopurulent cervicitis.

Bacterial vaginosis

■ Produces thin, grayish white discharge with fishy odor

Candida albicans infection

■ Produces thick, white, curdlike discharge with a yeastlike odor
■ Appears in patches on the cervix and vaginal walls

Causes of mucopurulent cervicitis

Chlamydia

Chlamydia is a common sexually transmitted disease caused by the organism *Chlamydia trachomatis.* Although 75% of women with chlamydia are asymptomatic, the disease may cause mucopurulent cervical discharge and cystitis.

Gonorrhea

Although gonorrhea commonly produces no symptoms, it may cause a purulent yellow discharge and cystitis.

Mucopurulent cervicitis

■ Produces purulent yellow discharge from the cervical os
■ Occurs with chlamydia and gonorrhea

Trichomoniasis

■ May produce a malodorous yellow or green, frothy or watery, foul-smelling discharge
■ May also involve red papules on the cervix and vaginal walls, giving the tissue a "strawberry" appearance

Genital warts

Genital warts, a sexually transmitted disease caused by human papillomavirus, produce painless warts on the vulva, vagina, cervix, or anus. Warts start as tiny red or pink swellings that grow and develop stemlike structures. Multiple swellings with a cauliflower appearance are common.

Genital warts on perineum

Genital herpes

Genital herpes produces multiple, shallow vesicles, lesions, or crusts inside the vagina, on the external genitalia, on the buttocks and, sometimes, on the thighs. Dysuria, regional lymph node inflammation, pain, edema, and fever may be present.

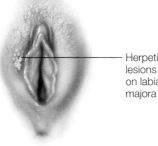

Herpetic lesions on labia majora

Vaginal and uterine prolapse

Also called *cystocele*, vaginal prolapse occurs when the anterior vaginal wall and bladder prolapse into the vagina. During speculum examination, you'll see a pouch or bulging on the anterior wall as the patient bears down. The uterus may prolapse into the vagina and even be visible outside the body.

Cystocele

Cervical polyps

Cervical polyps are bright red, soft, and fragile. They're typically benign, but they may bleed. They usually arise from the endocervical canal.

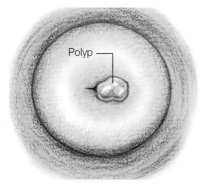

Polyp

Cervical cancer

During a speculum examination, you may detect hard, granular, friable lesions—signs of late-stage cervical cancer. In the early stages of cervical cancer, the cervix looks normal.

Ectocervical lesion

Rectocele

Rectocele is herniation of the rectum through the posterior vaginal wall. On examination, you'll see a pouch or bulging on the posterior wall as the patient bears down.

Rectocele

Male genital abnormalities

outside the norm

Common male genital lesions

Penile cancer

Penile cancer causes a painless, ulcerative lesion on the glans or prepuce (foreskin), possibly accompanied by discharge.

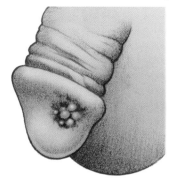

Genital herpes

Genital herpes causes a painful, reddened group of small vesicles or blisters on the prepuce, shaft, or glans. Lesions eventually disappear but tend to recur.

Genital warts

Genital warts are flesh-colored, soft, moist papillary growths that occur singly or in cauliflower-like clusters. They may be barely visible or several inches in diameter.

Syphilis

Syphilis causes a hard, round papule on the penis. When palpated, this syphilitic chancre may feel like a button. Eventually, the papule erodes into an ulcer. You may also note swollen lymph nodes in the inguinal area.

Testicular tumor

A painless scrotal nodule that can't be transilluminated may be a testicular tumor, which could be benign or cancerous. The tumor can grow, enlarging the testis.

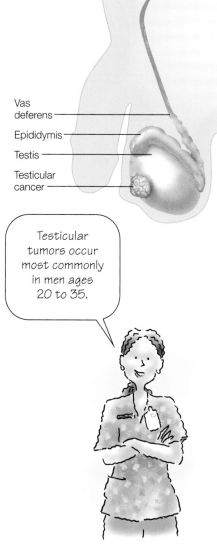

Vas deferens

Epididymis

Testis

Testicular cancer

Testicular tumors occur most commonly in men ages 20 to 35.

Prostate gland enlargement

A smooth, firm, symmetrical enlargement of the prostate gland indicates benign prostatic hyperplasia, which typically starts after age 50. This finding may be associated with nocturia, urinary hesitancy and frequency, and recurring urinary tract infections.

In acute prostatitis, the prostate gland is firm, warm, and extremely tender and swollen. Because bacterial infection causes the condition, the patient usually has a fever.

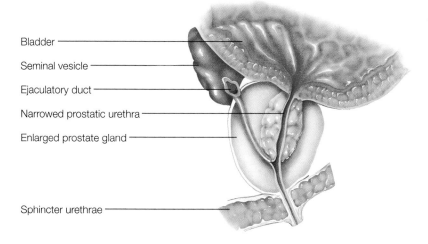

- Bladder
- Seminal vesicle
- Ejaculatory duct
- Narrowed prostatic urethra
- Enlarged prostate gland
- Sphincter urethrae

Prostate gland lesions

Hard, irregular, fixed lesions that make the prostate feel asymmetrical suggest prostate cancer. Palpation may be painful. This condition also causes urinary dysfunction. Back and leg pain may occur with bone metastases in advanced stages.

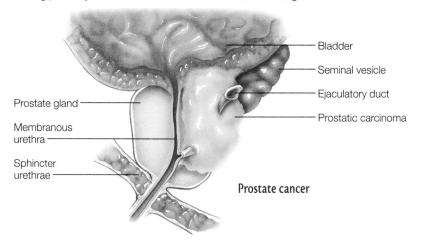

- Bladder
- Seminal vesicle
- Ejaculatory duct
- Prostatic carcinoma
- Prostate gland
- Membranous urethra
- Sphincter urethrae

Prostate cancer

Hernia

A hernia is the protrusion of an organ through an abnormal opening in the muscle wall. It may be direct or indirect, inguinal or femoral.

A direct inguinal hernia emerges from behind the external inguinal ring and protrudes through it. This type of hernia seldom descends into the scrotum and usually affects men older than age 40.

An indirect inguinal hernia is the most common type of hernia; it occurs in men of all ages. It can be palpated in the internal inguinal canal with its tip in or beyond the canal, or the hernia may descend into the scrotum.

Uncommon in men, a femoral hernia feels like a soft tumor below the inguinal ligament in the femoral area. It may be difficult to distinguish from a lymph node.

Inguinal hernia

VISION QUEST

Able to label?

Identify the structures of the male reproductive system indicated on this illustration.

1. _____
2. _____
3. _____

4. _____
5. _____

Rebus riddle

Sound out each group of pictures and symbols to reveal information about the urinary system.

The 🫘🫘 📋 ur + 🏨 Vacancies and maintain 🤸 of 🧴🧴🧴.

Answers: Able to label? 1. Seminal vesicles, 2. Vas deferens, 3. Prostate gland, 4. Urethra, 5. Epididymis; Rebus riddle: The kidneys form urine and maintain balance of fluids.

Selected references

Alcenius, M. "Successfully Meet Pain Assessment Standards," *Nursing Management* 35(3):12, March 2004.

Anatomy & Physiology Made Incredibly Easy, 2nd ed. Philadelphia: Lippincott Williams & Wilkins, 2005.

Assessment: An Incredibly Easy Pocket Guide. Philadelphia: Lippincott Williams & Wilkins, 2006.

Assessment Made Incredibly Easy, 3rd ed. Philadelphia: Lippincott Williams & Wilkins, 2005.

Bickley, L.S., and Szilagyi, P.G. *Bates' Guide to Physical Examination and History Taking*, 9th ed. Philadelphia: Lippincott Williams & Wilkins, 2007.

Coviello, J.S. "Cardiac Assessment 101: A New Look at the Guidelines for Cardiac Homecare Patients," *Home Healthcare Nurse* 22(2):116-23, February 2004.

Kasper, D.L., et al., eds. *Harrison's Principles of Internal Medicine*, 16th ed. New York: McGraw-Hill Book Co., 2005.

Potter, P.A., and Perry, A.G. *Fundamentals of Nursing*, 6th ed. St. Louis: Mosby–Year Book, Inc., 2005.

Professional Guide to Signs & Symptoms, 5th ed. Philadelphia: Lippincott Williams & Wilkins, 2007.

Pullen, R.L., Jr. "Neurologic Assessment for Pronator Drift," *Nursing2004* 34(3):22, March 2004.

Rhoads, J. *Advanced Health Assessment and Diagnostic Reasoning.* Philadelphia: Lippincott Williams & Wilkins, 2006.

Thibodeau, G.A., and Potter, K.T. *The Human Body in Health and Disease*, 4th ed. St. Louis: Mosby–Year Book, Inc., 2005.

Weber, J., and Kelley, J. *Health Assessment in Nursing*, 2nd ed. Philadelphia: Lippincott Williams & Wilkins, 2003.

Woodrow, P. "Assessing Blood Pressure in Older People," *Nursing Older People* 16(1):29-31, March 2004.

Woods, S.L., et al. *Cardiac Nursing*, 5th ed. Philadelphia: Lippincott Williams & Wilkins, 2005.

Credits

Chapter 1

David (Michelangelo), pages 1 and 2. Scala/Art Resource, NY.

Chapter 2

Freckles, page 15. From Goodheart, H.P., MD. *Goodheart's Photoguide of Common Skin Disorders*, 2nd ed. Philadelphia: Lippincott Williams & Wilkins, 2003.

Psoriasis, page 20. Sauer, G.C. *Manual of Skin Diseases*, 5th ed. Philadelphia: Lippincott, 1985.

Contact dermatitis, Urticaria, Herpes zoster, Scabies, Tinea corporis, pages 20 and 21. From Goodheart, H.P., MD. *Goodheart's Photoguide of Common Skin Disorders*, 2nd ed. Philadelphia: Lippincott Williams & Wilkins, 2003.

Alopecia, page 24. Image provided by Stedman's.

Hirsutism, page 24. From Goodheart, H.P., MD. *Goodheart's Photoguide of Common Skin Disorders*, 2nd ed. Philadelphia: Lippincott Williams & Wilkins, 2003.

Splinter hemorrhages, page 25. From Gold, D.H., MD, and Weingeist, T.A., MD, PhD. *Color Atlas of the Eye in Systemic Disease*. Baltimore: Lippincott Williams & Wilkins, 2001.

Terry's nails, page 25. Habif, T.P. *Clinical Dermatology: A Color Guide to Diagnosis and Therapy*, 2nd ed. St. Louis: C.V. Mosby, 1990.

Chapter 3

Mona Lisa (Leonardo da Vinci), pages 27 and 33. Réunion des Musées Nationaux/Art Resource, NY.

Queen Nefertiti, page 38. Bildarchiv Preussischer Kulturbesitz/Art Resource, NY.

Acute angle-closure glaucoma, Periorbital edema, pages 43 and 44. From Bickley, L.S., and Szilagyi, P. *Bates' Guide to Physical Examination and History Taking*, 8th ed. Philadelphia: Lippincott Williams & Wilkins, 2003.

Chapter 4

Structures of the neck, page 53. From Weber J., and Kelley, J. *Health Assessment in Nursing*, 2nd ed. Philadelphia: Lippincott Williams & Wilkins, 2003.

Herpes simplex, Angioedema, pages 60 and 61. From Neville, B., et al. *Color Atlas of Clinical Oral Pathology*. Philadelphia: Lea & Febiger, 1991.

Leukoplakia, Candidiasis, page 61. Robinson, H.B.G., and Miller, A.S. *Colby, Kerr, and Robinson's Color Atlas of Oral Pathology*. Philadelphia: J.B. Lippincott, 1990.

Tonsillitis, Pharyngitis, page 63. Wellcome Photo Library.

Diphtheria, page 63. Reproduced with permission from Harnisch, J.P., et al.: "Diphtheria among alcoholic urban adults," *Ann Intern Med* 111:77, 1989.

Chapter 7

Lobes and ducts, page 115. From Weber, J., and Kelley, J. *Health Assessment in Nursing*, 2nd ed. Philadelphia: Lippincott Williams & Wilkins, 2003.

The Birth of Venus (Sandro Botticelli), page 118. Scala/Art Resource, NY.

Gynecomastia, page 125. From Weber J., and Kelley, J. *Health Assessment in Nursing*, 2nd ed. Philadelphia: Lippincott Williams & Wilkins, 2003.

Chapter 8

Examining the rectum and anus, Gas, Tumor, Incisional hernia, pages 141 and 142. From Bickley, L.S., and Szilagyi, P. *Bates' Guide to Physical Examination and History Taking*, 8th ed. Philadelphia: Lippincott Williams & Wilkins, 2003.

Chapter 9

Heberden's nodes, Bouchard's nodes, page 167. © NMSB/Custom Medical Stock Photo.

Ganglion, page 167. From Weber, J., and Kelley, J. *Health Assessment in Nursing*, 2nd ed. Philadelphia: Lippincott Williams & Wilkins, 2003.

Gout, page 168. © NMSB/Custom Medical Stock Photo.

Chapter 10

Vitruvian Man (Leonardo da Vinci), page 183. Alinari/Art Resource, NY.

Pupils, page 189. From Bickley, L.S., and Szilagyi, P. *Bates' Guide to Physical Examination and History Taking*, 8th ed. Philadelphia: Lippincott Williams & Wilkins, 2003.

Inspecting the genitalia, Palpating Bartholin's glands, pages 199 and 200. From Weber, J., and Kelley, J. *Health Assessment in Nursing*, 2nd ed. Philadelphia: Lippincott Williams & Wilkins, 2003.

We gratefully acknowledge Anatomical Chart Company for the use of selected images.

Index